Psychology Revivals

New Dimensions of Deep Analysis

Originally published in 1954, *New Dimensions of Deep Analysis* was a systematic attempt at integrating facts which were once misrepresented as "occult" into the framework of modern dynamic psychiatry. Defining the concepts and criteria of so-called telepathic (or psi) phenomena, Dr Ehrenwald bases his discussion on a detailed analysis of a series of telepathic dreams observed in the psychoanalytic situation. These observations indicated that telepathy between analyst and patient, between mother and child – and in interpersonal relationships in general – was far more frequent and of much greater significance than was generally allowed for. Indeed, its very occurrence – described by the author as telepathic leakage – called for a revision and restatement of some of the classical propositions of psychoanalytic theory and practice, similar to that which had become necessary in the field of modern theoretical physics nearly half a century before. He redefines personality as an open *versus* a closed system made up of a three-fold stratification of ego-, id- and psi-levels. In his outline of what he describes as three-level therapy he tries to apply these concepts to the doctor-patient relationship and to come to grips with the magic element involved in the therapeutic process in accordance with established psychodynamic principles. Today it can be read in its historical context.

New Dimensions of Deep Analysis

A Study of Telepathy in Interpersonal Relationships

Jan Ehrenwald

Routledge
Taylor & Francis Group
LONDON AND NEW YORK

First published in 1954
by George Allen & Unwin Ltd

This edition first published in 2025 by Routledge
4 Park Square, Milton Park, Abingdon, Oxon, OX14 4RN

and by Routledge
605 Third Avenue, New York, NY 10017

Routledge is an imprint of the Taylor & Francis Group, an informa business

ISBN: 978-1-032-95454-7 (hbk)
ISBN: 978-1-003-58500-8 (ebk)
ISBN: 978-1-032-95457-8 (pbk)

Book DOI 10.4324/9781003585008

New Dimensions Of Deep Analysis

A STUDY OF TELEPATHY IN INTERPERSONAL RELATIONSHIPS

JAN EHRENWALD

M.D.

George Allen & Unwin Ltd

RUSKIN HOUSE · MUSEUM STREET · LONDON

First published in 1954

Printed in Great Britain
in 11-point Baskerville type
by Unwin Brothers Limited
Woking and London

Preface

IF the title chosen for this book suggests another presentation of psychoanalytic theory and practice—orthodox or unorthodox—the reader is likely to be disappointed. The chapters that follow are not intended to go once more over familiar territory and to elaborate on basic discoveries which have been revolutionary nearly half a century ago. These discoveries have by now become common ground to contemporary psychiatry and there is no new contribution to this field conceivable unless it builds on foundations laid by Freud and his school.

But the present study is not concerned with putting a new coat of paint on the structure erected by psychoanalysis nor with redecorating its interior in the taste of one or another of the dissenting schools. It is concerned with the description and psychodynamic evaluation of a new group of observations for which no provisions have been made in the main building of modern dynamic psychiatry and which urgently call for proper accommodation—if need be in a new wing or even in a new dimension of scientific thinking.

Strictly speaking, the observations are new only to our modern philosophical outlook. Usually described as psychical phenomena such as telepathy, clairvoyance, precognition or the like, they are relegated to the realm of folk-lore or superstition and are not accorded the status of factual scientific evidence deserving serious consideration. It is to avoid the stigma of primitive, pre-scientific thinking which is still attached to these concepts and to forestall preconceived ideas as to their nature that Professor R. H. Thouless and Dr. B. P. Wiesner* in England have suggested the Greek symbol *psi* for their designation. It is in this sense that the term will be used in the present study. There is only one preliminary assumption which cannot easily be avoided in adopting the term: the assumption that *psi* phenomena do in reality exist.

This assumption has indeed been made necessary by the

* See Bibliography.

vast mass of evidence which has accumulated in the past decades under both laboratory and spontaneous conditions—that is, in the familiar type of card-calling experiments developed by Professor J. B. Rhine and his associates, and in the less familiar observations recorded by a small group of psychiatrists and psychoanalysts in the psychotherapeutic situation.

This latter group of observations suggests that *psi* functions play an important part in man's mental organization. They are closely related to unconscious portions of the ego and super-ego and to what Freud has described as the *id,* and even though their existence is not usually accessible to conscious self-observation or, for that matter, to observation by ordinary clinical methods, they may have a significant effect upon interpersonal relationships in both health and disease.

The implications of *psi* as a new aspect of the human mind are so far-reaching that they call for a revision and restatement of a number of current assumptions and theoretical presuppositions regarding personality structure, mind-body relationship, cerebral localization, and the nature of our perceptual world in general. Failing such an attempt, telepathy and related occurrences would have to remain nothing but incomprehensible and freakish accidents on the "lunatic fringe" of our experience, outside the pale of a rational scientific scheme of thinking.

What, then, are the facts as they can be ascertained on applying the method of modern dynamic psychiatry to our issue? How can they be reconciled with our established body of experience regarding the working of the human mind? In what way, if any, can the newly found insight be utilized for a better understanding of the dynamics of psychoanalytic treatment and of interpersonal relationships in general?

These are some of the principal questions which will be discussed in the chapters that follow. Their discussion will be largely based on observations made by the present writer in the psychoanalytic situation. He cannot therefore claim more than the validity of simple clinical data in their behalf. They have no more (but also no less) objective validity than a patient's verbal account of a dream, a hallucination or an anxiety attack. Nevertheless, few will deny the justification of the psychiatrist's attempt at systematic investigation of such clinical data. The same right for an objective hearing is claimed for the observations described here.

It is true that many doubts have been raised as to the very possibility of *psi* phenomena. They are stated to be in flagrant contradiction to the established laws of nature. Their occurrence is said to be "intrinsically improbable." But that does not seem to preclude their actual occurrence. It is also true that their investigation under spontaneous conditions is beset with many difficulties, greater even than those encountered in laboratory tests concerned with extrasensory perception or ESP. But given an unbiased and flexible approach—one that does not try to prescribe the exact way in which the incidents observed are supposed to behave and that makes due allowance for the peculiar psychological constellation in which they are apt to occur—the ground seems to be cleared for their closer investigation. Indeed, the time may not be far away when it will be possible to predict their occurrence with the same degree of probability with which an experienced psychiatrist can predict the emergence of a particular type of dream, the reactivation of a delusional trend or of an anxiety symptom in his patients.

More will have to be said about the peculiar psychological constellation favourable to the emergence of *psi* phenomena. But three factors should be stressed from the outset. First, telepathy is more likely to occur in an atmosphere of social approval than in an atmosphere of doubt and disapprobation. Secondly, it is promoted by the existence of a more or less pronounced personal bond or *rapport* between those involved and, thirdly, by a heightened emotional tone or temperature prevailing in the total situation.

Critics have taken objection to this state of affairs. They have called for the demonstration of spontaneous occurrences under conditions which would be bound to defeat their spontaneity. They want them to materialize at the beck and call of a sceptical experimenter, armed with film camera and tape recorder, ready to observe but refusing to participate in terms of what H. S. Sullivan has called participant observation.

Yet their most vehement objection is levelled against the fact that certain emotionally coloured motivations on the part of those involved seem to be an indispensable prerequisite of the incidents. It is as though a chemist were called upon to demonstrate a chemical reaction but was strictly forbidden the use of a Bunsen burner because the flame might blacken his test tube.

There is no denying that conditions of observation meeting with those requirements are difficult to establish. The observer's participation may easily exceed the limits within which objective observation is feasible. Again, in the absence of his actual involvement and participation, nothing may be left for him to observe. But the case histories described in the first part of the present study show that, under favourable circumstances, a happy combination of the two seemingly conflicting attitudes can be achieved. This is further demonstrated by the recent publications of other psychiatrists and psychoanalysts pursuing a similar line. I may only mention the contributions of J. Eisenbud, G. Pederson-Krag, M. Ullman, J. Meerloo and G. Booth in the United States; of W. H. Gillespie and Alice E. Buck in England, E. Servadio in Italy, Tenhaeff in Holland, H. Bender in Germany and H. J. Urban in Austria.

Those living in the New York area joined in 1947 in an informal research group and formed a Medical Section of the American Society for Psychical Research. Since then they have reported a great many incidents of the kind discussed here. This seems to indicate that it is the community of purpose and scientific curiosity animating the members of the group that has, against all odds inherent in our culture, helped to create the very intellectual and emotional climate which, as I said, is indispensable for the occurrences. It is therefore to the members of the New York group and to the stimulation and encouragement received from them that I want to express my feelings of gratitude in the first place. To this I must add thanks to Mrs. Laura A. Dale of the American Society for Psychical Research and to my wife for the invaluable help they have given me in the preparation of this book. I am also greatly indebted to Professor Gardner Murphy and Dr. Montague Ullman for their constructive criticism and comments. Last but not least I have to thank my patients upon whose case studies the major part of the present book is based and who have consented to their publication. They will find that personal references have been considerably disguised so as to ensure their anonymity. I wish to emphasize, however, that all accounts of actual telepathic incidents and their surrounding circumstances—including those involving myself—have remained unchanged. Their description is based on verbatim records taken during the analytic session and conveys "the truth and nothing but the truth," as it presented itself to the present writer—even where he could not help "incriminating" himself by submitting it for publication. This, however, is a professional risk incurred by any author engaged in such an unorthodox field of research as that concerned with the nature of *psi* phenomena.

New York, Spring 1952

Acknowledgements

SPECIAL thanks are due to the Editors of the *American Journal for Psychotherapy; Psychiatric Quarterly* and *Psychoanalytic Review* for permission to reprint substantial parts of articles previously published in their Journals. They are specifically referred to in footnotes to the text. I also wish to thank the *Creative Age Press* (Mrs. Eileen Garrett) for permission to reproduce Fig. 2 on page 12 from Warcollier's book *Mind to Mind* (New York, 1948).

Contents

PART THREE: *Can it be Applied in Practice? An Approach to Therapy*

Illustrations

Tables

PART ONE

TELEPATHY IN THE PSYCHOANALYTIC SITUATION

A REVIEW OF ILLUSTRATIVE CASES

Have I given you the impression that I am secretly inclined to support the reality of telepathy in the occult sense? If so, I should very much regret that it is so difficult to avoid giving such an impression.

FREUD, 1922

When such things as telepathic messages do exist, we cannot rule out the possibility that they reach the sleeper and may be grasped by him. Nay, judging from the analogy with such other materials as sensory impressions and thought processes we must assume that telepathic messages, received in the waking state, might be registered in the succeeding night.

FREUD, 1925

I am convinced you will be rather dissatisfied with my attitude toward this problem: not fully convinced yet ready to be convinced. Maybe you will say to yourself: There you have another instance of a man who after a life's work as a respectable scientist is becoming demented or gullible in his ripe old age.

FREUD, 1933

CHAPTER I

Operational Concepts and Guiding Principles

THE old saying that today's heresy may turn out to be tomorrow's commonplace has to be taken with a grain of salt. Today's heretic may conceivably be exposed as tomorrow's fool. Again, the fallacies and superstitions of a past age may re-emerge from the scientific limbo and claim their rightful place among the respectable scientific disciplines of a new era.

Is the heresy of a new dynamic psychology, based on the proper appreciation of telepathy and related phenomena, destined to become the psychology of tomorrow, or is it a throwback to the pre-scientific, magic and animistic beliefs of our ancestors?

Only the systematic exposition of such a thesis and its methodical application to all the facts and facets of our up-to-date knowledge concerning the human mind will give the answer. The chapters that follow are intended as an attempt at such a systematic exposition. They will take the existence of *psi* functions for granted—not because the evidence in their favour has ceased to be controversial, but because the continued amassing of further evidence alone is unlikely to settle the controversy one way or the other. What is needed is a consistent system of explanatory hypotheses, a coherent theory which helps us to understand, to digest and to organize the new and disturbing observations within our current system of thought. Once this is accomplished we need no longer waste time and effort in wearing down the emotional resistance of the sceptic and can go ahead with the task of rounding out our picture and integrating the newly acquired insight with our existing knowledge of the universe.

In an earlier book[32] I have tried to assemble the available evidence with a view of offering a working hypothesis about the part played by telepathy and related phenomena in our everyday life in both health and disease.

It may be well to make some of the formulations presented there the point of departure in the present context. Most of the evidence reviewed made it clear that telepathy is a primitive, uncontrollable means of communication from one person to another. It cannot be "willed" in the way I can turn my head to the right or left or bend my index finger. Telepathy is not amenable to deliberate volition. More often than not it happens when we least expect it to occur and it fails to materialize whenever we seek to bring it about to order, as it were.

The occurrence of telepathy seems to be facilitated by a number of predisposing factors, mental or physical, on the part of the so-called agent and the so-called percipient. Among such factors, operating on the part of the percipient, a certain relaxed, passive attitude, resulting in freedom from inner tension has been widely accepted. In many cases what I described as *minus functions* of the ego, global or circumscribed, organic or functional, lasting or transient, were found responsible for telepathic sensitiveness. These observations, supported by a few striking cases in which such minus functions seemed to correspond with unusual telepathic abilities precisely in the sphere of an existing defect, led to the formulation of the *compensation theory* of telepathic sensitiveness on the part of the percipient.

However, it will be well to realize that such a theory seeks to account for the phenomena largely in physiological or structural terms, much in the same way as the neurologist tries to explain an aphasic reaction of his patient in terms of organic brain damage, leaving psychodynamic factors out of the picture. Yet it should be recalled that even in cases of this type the patient's repressed wishes and expectations may play an important part.

As far as the agent is concerned, Freud[44] has pointed to certain characteristics of the former's mental attitude. In the cases that had come to his notice Freud suggested that it is the emotionally charged preconscious or unconscious ideas which are apt to assume telepathic activity in the mind of an agent, ideas, that is to say, in their transitional state from the preconscious into the conscious sphere. Among the factors which have emerged from experimental studies, J. B. Rhine,[103] Gardner Murphy[86] and their associates place great emphasis on the spontaneity bordering on a playful attitude of both agent and percipient—provided that they are motivated by the desire that the experiment be a success. That motivations of this kind need not necessarily coincide with conscious goal-directed attitudes goes without saying. Experiments carried out by Gertrude Schmeidler[111] at the City College of New York, have shown, furthermore, that other things being equal, subjects assuming a positive attitude toward the possibility of *psi*-occurrences are more likely to score in excess of chance expectation than sceptics and disbelievers.

In this way we arrive at two complementary sets of predisposing factors, one concerning the agent, the other concerning the percipient. On the part of the agent we find pronounced emotional charge of certain ideas, thoughts or complexes, more often than not brought about by repression, total or partial, of the material concerned. On the part of the percipient it is all the factors amounting to a minus function, as described above, which may, under otherwise favourable conditions, be conducive to telepathy.

Yet the concept of compensation, as applied here, is also in need of qualification. The old thesis that the organism is able to make up for the loss of one specific function by hyperfunction in another sphere has rightly been subjected to criticism, e.g. by Kurt Goldstein[51] and the Gestalt psychologists. We have rather to assume that it is the effort of the total personality which is capable of "compensating" for any loss of ability within a special performance field. In short, the concept of compensation has to be substituted by a changed level of functioning which may, however, be interpreted in terms of a successful compensation on the part of the organism concerned.

It goes without saying that these formulations are of a purely heuristic nature and give but an incomplete picture of the real facts. Whoever is using them as operational concepts has to realize that neither an existing minus function nor the presence of a certain emotional charge of a given set of ideas is sufficient to bring about a telepathic incident as a matter of course. Another predisposing factor involved in many, though not all, cases is the presence of a more or less direct personal bond or *rapport* between agent and percipient. Telepathy does not come about with the same regularity with which a safety match ignites whenever it strikes a suitably prepared surface. It does not work like a chemical reaction once all the requisite ingredients are brought together in a test tube. Gardner Murphy[86] has pointed out that wherever we succeed in throwing light upon the psychodynamics of a given telepathic incident we find that it answers some emotional need of either the agent or the percipient. This point has specifically been emphasized by Jule Eisenbud[33] and will further be borne out by the material discussed in the chapters that follow. Reverting to the metaphor of a chemical reaction, telepathy seems to require a certain optimal emotional temperature, failing which the reaction does not come about. Indeed, I hinted in the Preface that its emergence is largely dependent on a certain cultural climate, on a specific situational context which favours its occurrence instead of penalizing the persons involved with ridicule or social ostracism.

This leads us to the question of certain specific personality traits which may or may not be detected in persons prone to telepathic experiences. Clinical evidence supplying clues in that direction will be discussed in Chapter XXI. More recently promising attempts at studying personalities apt to score in excess of chance expectation in ESP tests were made by B. M. Humphrey using the Elkisch personality test.[58] Her results indicate that the so-called extratensive personality types are more successful subjects in ESP experiments than the so-called introversive or constricted types.

As far as structural characteristics are concerned, a number of basic features of the telepathic material has emerged. Apart from a few spectacular occurrences in which the organization or Gestalt character of the material has been well preserved, telepathic experiences show all the qualities of unconscious mental content, such as the tendency to symbolic representation, condensation, displacement and secondary elaboration known from the imagery of the dream and the structure of the neurotic symptom. In these circumstances it is readily understood that the language spoken by the telepathic "message" is vague and equivocal, like the utterances of the Delphic Oracles. Telepathy rarely calls a spade a spade—or even an agricultural implement. It uses circumlocutions, it resorts to metaphors, to indirect and sometimes far-fetched allusions in the manner of the riddles and charades of a bygone age or of the picture puzzles of modern times.

In many spontaneous occurrences such as can be observed in everyday life, in dreams and in the psychoanalytic situation, telepathic correspondence of two contemporary mental events is suggested without reference to the exact physical nature or quality of the items concerned. In many instances it is the correlation which exists between the whole and the part, between a distinct idea and an apparently far-fetched association connected with it which is suggestive of telepathy. In these cases telepathy does not amount to a faithful reproduction of a distinct feature in another person's mind. It breaks it up into pieces, it suppresses one of its constituent parts and brings out another, it shifts the emphasis from the essential to the accidental, from the centre to the periphery, from the real thing to its symbolic representation, from the trivial to the preposterous—if not from the sublime to the ridiculous—like the rhyming slang of the cockney.

This is what I described as the scatter tendency of telepathic occurrences. It will be seen on a later page that this scatter effect is not confined to the dimension of space but also refers to the temporal aspect of the telepathic process, usually described in terms of postcognitive[18] or precognitive telepathy, or as the displacement effect discovered by W. Carington and confirmed by S. G. Soal and K. M. Goldney.[118]

All these manifest shortcomings of the telepathic function as a means of communication have served to deepen the suspicion of both the scientific world and the educated public toward it. Apart from contradicting all the established laws of nature, most accounts of spontaneous occurrences were vitiated by their vagueness and ambiguous nature, by the lack of contemporary written records or of reliable witnesses to testify to their authenticity. To make matters worse, the virtual impossibility of duplicating occasional successful experiments with so-called freely chosen material such as were used in Frederic Myers's drawing tests[87] had to be explained by a variety of auxiliary hypotheses.

These inadequacies of what psychical research describes as spontaneous evidence resulted in its ultimate rejection as a source of valid scientific data. This is why almost twenty-five years ago Professor J. B. Rhine and his associates at Duke University[103a] resorted to a new approach. Following earlier attempts by Richet,[104] Brugmans,[15] Estabrooks,[36] Ina Jephson[63] and others they devised the now familiar ESP tests and worked out methods of their statistical evaluation. These experiments, by focusing attention upon such simple data as the symbols printed on the Zener cards, eliminated most of the pitfalls attached to the study of such highly complex incidents as may occur in everyday life. At the same time they made exact mathematical treatment of results possible.

The new approach seemed to be the answer to the prayers of the worker in psychical research. It held the promise of making his endeavours at long last scientifically "respectable" and allowed him to dispense with all anecdotal accounts of occasional striking incidents upon which he had had to rely in the past. Like his colleagues in the neighbouring fields of clinical, social, and animal psychology, he could base his work on repeatable experiments under limited but well-controlled laboratory conditions.

Viewed against a broader historical background, the new fledgling branch of parapsychology thus reflects the cleavage which has existed in psychology at large long before modern dynamic psychiatry and the configurationist school had challenged the position of the nineteenth-century Wundtian laboratory approach. Then it was the "brick and mortar" concept of elementary sensory perceptions, associations of ideas, etc., versus the study of the total personality of man within his cultural context. Today it is the problem of the assumed telepathic transmission of isolated sensory impressions or mental images versus analytic inquiry into the psychodynamics of a given spontaneous incident within an existing social situation.

However, we should do well to realize that the gulf between the two types of phenomena is largely artificial. It is due to preconceived ideas about the apparent simplicity of the psychological problems involved in the ESP type of experiment on the one hand, and the greater complexity of spontaneous occurrences encountered in everyday life and in the psychoanalytic situation on the other.

It is true that occurrences of the latter type are of a more patently emotional nature than the former. Love, hatred, and the mortal crises of distant friends and relations are the principal themes of the cases described by Gurney, Myers and Podmore in their classic *Phantasms of the Living*.[52] We will see that similar *motifs* can be found at the bottom of observations derived from the psychoanalytic situation. In contrast, all the materials used in laboratory ESP experiments are of a seemingly trivial nature. At least it is assumed that such symbols as the circle, the star, the wavy lines, the cross, and the square which are reproduced on Dr. Rhine's Zener cards are devoid of any appreciable emotional appeal to the subject. Moreover, it seems to be readily understood that the usually quick succession of calls and the monotony of the whole procedure is not likely to stimulate the subject's interest. Yet I have pointed out elsewhere[32] that sensory material even of the most indifferent kind may well assume some emotional significance to a given subject. It may be derived either from the subject's past experience, from fleeting moods at the time of the experiment, or from the social context within which he finds himself in relation to the experimenter and his associates.

I have illustrated this point by a simple test. A number of subjects were asked to glance at one of the Zener cards and to tell me their impressions. A patient of mine, a lady of forty-six, was shown the five squares. She exclaimed: "Oh, they are like a repulsive face staring at me!" In a similar vein, the wavy lines reminded her of "disgusting little worms." A child of seven associated the five crosses with kisses in a letter, whilst her mother found that they reminded her of the melancholy array of soldiers' graves. There were other subjects whose associations were less imaginative and colourful. But the few reactions of the imaginative type are sufficient to show that even such trivial items as geometrical figures, wavy lines or plus signs, may call forth a wealth of emotionally coloured imagery in suitable subjects. The vast body of experience derived from the Rorschach test points in the same direction.

One could say that the psychodynamic factors which we assume are involved in experiments of the ESP type duplicate on a microscopical scale, as it were, the factors which can be revealed macroscopically by the psychoanalytic approach. It is this hypothesis combining, on the one hand, the postulate of a compensated minus function and the tendency to seek gratification of deep-seated emotional needs on the other, which forms the bridge between the two principal kinds of evidence upon which modern parapsychology is based.

Reverting to the simile about the match that ignites only when striking a suitably prepared rough surface, one could say that the requisite combination of favourable factors on the part of both agent and percipient are only rarely met with under laboratory conditions. This may account for the capricious distribution pattern of hits and misses in quantitative research. On the other hand, Rhine[103a] has pointed out that such well-known psychological and physiological factors as flagging of interest or fatigue may be responsible for the so-called decline effect resulting in the characteristic patterns of scores in both short runs and long-term series of card calling tests. It is precisely this unmistakable decline effect which has been invoked as a decisive argument against the chance explanation of the results—quite apart from the statistical significance of the total scores in successful subjects.

Nevertheless, in view of the capricious nature of experimental ESP scores a vast number of tests is required in order to obtain statistically significant results. This can be contrasted with the closer investigation of an individual case which may afford such a wealth of specific psychologically significant data as to enable us to dispense with the criterion of statistical significance. It will be seen that "good" telepathic incidents of this type are of a distinctly meaningful nature which can best be revealed by psychoanalytic inquiry into the personalities of the agent and percipient.

It goes without saying that no such inquiry can be applied

to an individual guess within a large series of card calling tests. The laboratory approach is unlikely to yield any fruitful information as to why Tom, Dick or Harry scored two or three extra-chance hits on a circle or square in the first run and failed to do so in the second or third. Here, as in many other fields of research, statistics say a little about a lot—whilst the individual approach says a lot about a little. One could say: The trawler net may be a practical device to catch an unspecified type of fish in great numbers, but when we set out to catch a particular rare specimen we have to resort to more sophisticated and more individualistic methods of fishing.

CHAPTER II

Psychological versus Statistical Significance

A Digression into Method

so far our account of operational concepts and guiding principles has left one important question out of the picture: What is the nature of the principal data upon which our formulations are based? What are the respective merits and shortcomings of the statistical evidence to which we have referred and how does this material compare with what we described as spontaneous evidence? I hinted that modern parapsychology has shown a definite preference for experimental data and their statistical evaluation. This is documented by the pioneer work of J. B. Rhine[103a, b, c] and his associates in the United States, and of G. N. M. Tyrrell,[131] S. G. Soal, and K. M. Goldney[118] and others in England.

Rhine and his followers took as their point of departure the assumed transmission, in some extrasensory way, of well-defined perceptual images or sensory impressions. They deliberately confined themselves to a single track along which their experiments were to proceed. Using the now familiar pack of Zener cards, they made the subject comply with the predetermined laboratory situation, that is, guess at one of the five symbols contained in the pack of twenty-five, carefully recording his scores and excluding all possibilities of sensory leakage, collusion or clerical errors. Hundreds of thousands of tests carried out under varying conditions indeed yielded results which authorities in the mathematics of probability have acclaimed as significant. There is fairly general agreement that the results arrived at in a sufficient number of long-term experiments were so far in excess of chance expectation that the odds against chance could only be expressed by astronomical figures. For example the anti-chance probability in the famous Soal–Goldney experiments with Basil Shackleton amounts to 10^{35}. This figure was even exceeded in Dr. Soal's[118a] more recent experiments with Mrs. Stewart. Again, the odds against chance in the earlier Pratt–Woodruff[96] experiments at Duke University were found to be 10^{14} to one. Professor R. H. Thouless[129] has pointed out that in order to arrive at such results by mere trial and error a larger number of experiments would be required than the whole history of the world allows for.

However, there is no denying that despite the accumulation of a vast mass of experimental data during the past decades little information about the *modus operandi* of *psi* functions has emerged. The laboratory approach, with all the ingenious variations of technique and experimental conditions, has failed to give an answer as to the nature of *psi* phenomena, as to the personality needs they fulfil and has certainly supplied no clues as to the psychodynamics involved. There can be little doubt that in this respect it shares the shortcomings of the quantitative statistical methods in general.

The need for proper appreciation of specific personality factors is amply illustrated by the published experimental observations themselves. A typical example which will be discussed in more detail in later pages may illustrate the point. Little Bo, a mentally defective child, scored far in excess of chance expectation in ESP tests carried out by Dr. Drake of Wesleyan College in Georgia. Yet Bo did so only with his mother playing the part of an agent and failed whenever other persons took her place in the experiment. Clearly, any explanation ascribing this state of affairs to nothing but chance is hardly tenable. It fails to account for the fact that the "chance results" were confined to two subjects tied together by a particular bond or *rapport*: the child-mother relationship.

Likewise, S. G. Soal,[118a] in his experiments with Mrs. Stewart in London, showed that his subject scored persistently above chance with certain agents only, whilst she failed to do so with other agents. Her scores dropped even when she was unaware of the fact that her favourite agent had been replaced by another. Many examples of the same kind can be quoted from the literature. They show that failing to pay due attention to the dynamics of interpersonal relationships involved in every experiment would seriously hamper the statistical evaluation of results if not altogether defeat its purpose.

There is another disadvantage that goes with a onesided laboratory approach. Confining our attention to such material as geometrical figures, numbers, letters of the alphabet, etc., we may be led to the unwarranted conception that paranormal cognition (or whatever it may be called) is really concerned with a quasi-sensory perception of elementary sense data, dehydrated, deboned, and filleted, as it were, for the convenience of the research worker. This idea has not been borne out by the facts. It is tenable only so long as we confine ourselves to simplified quantifiable material. Whenever we abandon the single-tracked laboratory method we light upon phenomena of an entirely different complexion, difficult to reconcile with the strictly mathematical approach.

What method other than that of statistical evaluation can, then, be applied in order to ascertain the extrasensory nature of such individual incidents?

In the present connection we are chiefly concerned with the problem of telepathy. As a general rule telepathy is assumed to be responsible for such similarity or correspondence of two simultaneous mental events which cannot be accounted for by chance, sensory leakage, or past common experiences of those involved. But what are the criteria of the similarity or correspondence of the two sets of "simultaneous" mental events upon which the assumption of their telepathic nature is based?

The early workers in psychical research, chiefly concerned as they were with the accumulation of facts, failed to give a satisfactory answer to this question. They laid down certain general rules which had to be observed in collecting the material. They agreed on certain postulates, failing which they dismissed the evidential value of a given case. But their rules were of a largely empirical nature derived from an essentially phenomenological approach and their evaluation based on intuition or common-sense judgments which, as Dr. Rhine[103] has pointed out, are bound to vary with the common sense—or bias—of those making judgments. This was precisely the reason why Dr. Rhine decided to restrict the use of spontaneous material as a source of scientific proof and to replace it with the study of quantifiable data and their statistical assessment.

Yet there is a number of criteria upon which research dealing with spontaneous material of a non-quantifiable nature can be based. These criteria can be summarized as follows: First, the elements or *motifs* which we assume are reproduced in a telepathic way must be identifiable as distinct elements within the context reviewed. Failing this, the claim of their supposed telepathic correspondence cannot be substantiated and indeed no further argument is possible.

Secondly, the element or *motif* thus defined must be of such a unique kind that its simultaneous appearance in the two presumably corresponding sets of mental events cannot reasonably be ascribed to chance. If I dream on a particular night that my schoolmate John Smith (and not just any John Smith known by that name) has met with a fatal accident on an icy road and if it can later be ascertained that this particular event has actually taken place in the described circumstances on the same night, and if I never had a similar dream before, the chance objection can reasonably be ruled out. We can then base our telepathic interpretation of the dream on the criterion of the *uniqueness* of the telepathic element concerned.

It is true that in practice only extremely rare observations are likely to be found which meet this criterion of uniqueness. More often than not the *motif* in question may at best show such a multiplicity of distinctive features as to leave little doubt as to its specificity in the two corresponding sets of mental events. In such a case their identification will be based on a process of "matching" similar to that used by the police for the apprehension of a person wanted for crime. If the picture of the person wanted shows sufficient resemblance with the person caught they are satisfied with his identity. This is not a method foolproof in the mathematical sense, but good enough as a practical procedure. It can, moreover, be supplemented by matching the fingerprints of the suspect—a device which is not, unfortunately, available in dealing with telepathic phenomena.

This is why even our broader formulations of the criterion of uniqueness or specificity leave many ambiguous cases of telepathic correspondence on our hands. I pointed out in the introductory remarks that the percipient rarely scores a direct telepathic hit on the agent's central idea, that his impression does not amount to a photographic replica of the "original." Indeed, I described the tendency to telepathic scatter as a basic characteristic of the process. Nevertheless, in a number of cases falling in this group the vague, nondescript material may carry with it some specific distinctive feature or identification tag, as it were, which may help in establishing its telepathic nature. The same principle is applied in modern biochemical experiments in which certain molecules are tagged with a so-called radioactive tracer element, easily detectable with the Geiger counter. The presence of such specific distinctive features in our cases may therefore be described as the psychological *tracer effect*. It can then be used as another criterion of the assumed telepathic correspondence.

A third and perhaps most important criterion is of an altogether different nature. In the chapter that follows I will discuss in more detail the dream of a patient featuring an apartment whose description showed a striking resemblance to my own, into which I had moved a few days before the dream occurred. The dreamer listed a number of distinctive features of the apartment. She described its layout and furnishings and prepared a drawing to substantiate her account. She could not have learned of these details by any conceivable sensory means. Nevertheless, it might well be objected that the assumed resemblance between my apartment and the one seen by the dreamer is a matter of degree and that therefore the weight which is to be attached to the criterion of specificity of the elements contained in the manifest dream content is open to debate.

Yet when the telepathic interpretation of the apartment *motif* featured in the dream was introduced into its psychoanalytic setting the whole dream suddenly appeared in a new light. Apparently meaningless before, it now became evident that it expressed the patient's unconscious desire to move into the therapist's home and to be adopted as a daughter by her father substitute. In short, the telepathic interpretation threw new light on the transference relationship, and made otherwise unintelligible details of the dream fall into a pattern: it was psychologically significant. It is this criterion of *psychological significance* which may serve as an important *added* criterion to the telepathic nature of an actual incident.

On reviewing the considerable number of spontaneous telepathic incidents that have been observed in the psycho-analytic situation in recent years, it will be noted that in most cases it is just this added insight into psychodynamics which not only justifies but indeed calls for a telepathic interpretation. This, for instance, is the case in the recent observations of Jule Eisenbud,[33a,b,c,] Geraldine Pederson-Krag,[93] N. Fodor,[38] M. Ullman,[133] Joost Meerloo[81] and W. H. Gillespie.[53a]

It is true that in all these observations the criterion of psychological significance is only tacitly implied as a guiding principle and chief emphasis is laid on the psychodynamic appraisal of the evidence. It may well be that it is this failure to clarify concepts and to define criteria—unavoidable in pioneer work—which has invited the attacks launched by Dr. Albert Ellis[34] in the *Psychiatric Quarterly* especially against Dr. Eisenbud[33] and his associates. This is not the place to go into the details of the Ellis–Eisenbud controversy but a few points call for comment in the present context. Dr. Ellis insists that the evidence afforded by Eisenbud is flimsy, far-fetched and amenable to a variety of non-telepathic interpretations, each of them equally pertinent. His second objection refers to the unmistakable emotional charge the issue of telepathy seems to evoke in those involved in the incidents. In Ellis's view observations made under such conditions are inconsistent with the scientific method: an emotional attitude assumed by the observer may easily cloud his judgment and falsify results. That is to say, Dr. Ellis calls for an experimental setting which, from all we know about the factors favouring the occurrence of telepathy, would promptly result in its obliteration.

In a subsequent article Ellis[34] goes one step further. He seeks to show in a facetious manner that using Eisenbud's method of interpretation, the occurrence of telepathy can be demonstrated in any parallel series of mental events pertaining to an alleged agent and an alleged percipient. To do this he chooses pairs of personalities assumed to be related in a telepathic way. Yet in order to demonstrate the absurdity of the telepathy hypothesis his choice is persons linked together by a purely fictitious bond. More than that: as one of his examples he picks the thoughts and emotions of the hero of Stewart Engstrand's *The Sling and the Arrow*, published in 1947, and argues the case of their hypothetical telepathic correspondence with one of the dreams described by Eisenbud at about the same time. No one will be surprised that Ellis, by disregarding the criterion of psychological consistency as described here—and by accepting the flimsiest of formal resemblances at their face value—succeeds in exposing the fallacies inherent in such a procedure. But in trying to prove his point Ellis only brings into sharper focus the need for paying due attention to the criteria outlined here.

The importance of the criterion of psychological significance to the whole issue under review calls for a brief digression into its nature. Clearly, if it is claimed that the telepathic interpretation, for instance, of a dream, is meaningful—that is to say, psychologically significant—it may rightly be asked in what way we arrive at such a conclusion. The answer is that it must fit in with what Bertrand Russell[108] described as a "consistent system of rational beliefs in which each part lends support to every other part" and thus attains a certain degree of credibility of its own.

A brief reflection on the way by which psychoanalysis has arrived at its system of thought should throw more light on this aspect of our problem. Freud,[44a] in his interpretation of the Oedipus myth, indicated the growing boy's longing for the sole possession of his mother as its dominating theme. This desire, he submits, carries in itself the seed of self-imposed punishment culminating in the supreme ordeal of symbolic castration. Freud described the Oedipus myth as the nuclear conflict of all neuroses and his findings were confirmed by his followers in a great number of clinical observations. We know now that Hamlet's inability to take vengeance on his villainous uncle is nothing but a variation on the same theme. Likewise, certain initiation rites seen in pre-literate peoples amounting to the symbolic castration of their adolescents become intelligible in the light of the Oedipus complex. So is a wide variety of dreams, fairy tales, social customs and institutions as well as works of art in many civilizations in many historic periods. Findings like these have firmly established the important part played by this complex in man's unconscious motivations in both health and disease. The discovery of the Oedipus complex thus brought order into chaos. It proved to be meaningful or psychologically significant in the broadest sense.

The same principle has paved the way for a growing body of analytical insight into many and varied facets of human behaviour. Freud,[44b] seeking to unravel the hidden meaning of a slip of the tongue, of a joke, of an apparently indifferent element in the manifest content of a dream or of a neurotic symptom, persistently sought to fit it in with the general context of his system of thought and with the prevailing scientific *Weltanschauung* of his time.

Comparing Freud's basic approach with the methods used by the dissenting schools of psychoanalysis, it is obvious that they applied the same guiding principles. For Alfred Adler[2] it is the consistency with the patient's style of life which serves as the principal criterion of a dynamic understanding of his symptom. For C. G. Jung[65] it is the operation of a repressed complex in its relationship to the individual and collective unconscious. In short, whatever be the specific type of interpretation offered, it is ultimately determined by the principle of psychological significance or consistency with Bertrand Russell's "overall system of rational beliefs" rooted in the prevailing scientific outlook of our culture.

One might expect that applying this criterion should be a perfectly legitimate method of reasoning in the field of psychology at large. Yet, while we see that modern dynamic psychology is indeed fully satisfied with the validity of its own non-quantifiable, interpretative approach, it demands a totally different standard of scientific proof as soon as it is confronted with observations which go beyond its established body of experience.

The orthodox analyst may not hesitate to interpret a certain element contained in the manifest content of a dream in terms of meaningful relationships with the dreamer's past experiences. But he will in all probability reject the identical interpretation if it is based on equally meaningful relationships with some other person's experiences, past or present, with whom the dreamer happens to be in telepathic *rapport*.

Why, then, should two different standards be applied to what appears to be basically the same clinical material? Elsewhere[32] I discussed in more detail the emotional aspects of the resistance of both scientist and educated layman to the telepathy hypothesis. But it may be well to realize at this point that this resistance is not of purely emotional origin. There can be little doubt that in trying to fit telepathy into our current system of thought we are faced with a genuine logical difficulty. It will be recalled that our definition of psychological significance is based on the criterion of consistency of a proposed telepathic interpretation with an overall system of rational beliefs *current* in an existing culture. Now there is no use denying the apparent inconsistency of *psi* phenomena with our current beliefs, deemed to be rational. The fact is that the notion of telepathy, of action at a distance, of "mind over matter," and all it implies, is in flagrant contradiction to our familiar system of thought. We stated that all the evidence that can be marshalled in its favour is at best of a statistical nature, supported by a few freakish observations meeting with the criterion of uniqueness. So-called spontaneous evidence, until now, has remained more than controversial precisely because any new system of thought which includes *psi* phenomena within its frame of reference (and which has to be resorted to in support of their validity) undoubtedly is in conflict with our prevailing concepts.

Clearly, we are caught at this point in the web of circular reasoning. The great majority of purportedly telepathic observations cannot be proved to be telepathic because telepathy is considered to be in conflict with our established system of thought. On the other hand, there is no reason to adjust our system of thought to the occurrence of telepathic phenomena because it is claimed that there are too few verifiable data available to warrant such an adjustment. This is how one might be led to the conclusion that the occurrence of telepathy is not amenable to other than statistical proof and cannot be the legitimate concern of dynamically oriented psychology or psychiatry.

There is only one way out of this vicious circle. We have to admit the validity of data based on the criterion of psychological significance in a tentative way—irrespective of their conflict with our preconceived ideas. The proof of the pudding will then be exclusively in the eating. That is, we will have to show that the introduction of the telepathic factor into a revised and expanded system of dynamic psychiatry does in actual fact result in a new rational system of thought, more inclusive than, and therefore preferable to, the old system. No doubt, such a revised and expanded system of dynamic psychiatry can enfold only step by step as more and more corroborative evidence comes to our notice.

To sum up, the study of telepathy and related phenomena has to be guided by three criteria on which the validity of our

Group	Data	Method	Criteria	Nature of Material
I	Quantifiable material, e.g. Rhine's card-calling tests	Mathematical assessment, probability calculation	Statistical significance	Quantifiable
II	Names, dates, numerals, combination of distinctive features	Phenomenological description, authentication of evidence	Uniqueness, "tracer effect"	Cognitive, ideational, unequivocal
III	Meaningful relationships, "intelligible constellations" (Kardiner)	Psychoanalytic; "comparative analysis" of agent and percipient	Psychological significance, consistency	Symbolic distorted, largely preconscious

Table I

The Roman figures (horizontal rows) indicate three types of evidence or scientific data on which research into telepathy can be based. The vertical columns indicate the principal characteristics of the data.

data can be based. First, by the criterion of statistical significance, provided that the data are amenable to the mathematical method. This is illustrated by Dr. Rhine's card-calling experiments. Secondly, by the criterion of uniqueness or specificity, provided that the incident in question contains material of such exceptional kind (names, dates, numbers or a combination of other identifying data) that chance can be ruled out without resort to the mathematical method. Material of this kind has been afforded by the early workers in psychical research. Thirdly, the argument may be based on the criterion of psychological significance or consistency with a rational system of beliefs such as are being held within a given cultural pattern. It will be seen that a great part of the evidence which is discussed in the chapters that follow falls into this third group but is supported by criteria of the second type.

It goes without saying that few observations will be of such a nature as to do justice to all three criteria just described. Each case has to be judged on its own merits and its evaluation must be based on the criterion of calculable probability, on the presence of tracer effects and on the evidence of psychological significance contained in the material.

CHAPTER III

*Ruth's Telepathic Dream**

IF the reader has ever taken a walk along the sandy beach of the seashore he may have come across an empty bottle washed ashore by the ocean. If he took a second look at the bottle he may have noticed that the bottle was corked. And he may well find that the same is true for all bottles which happen to be washed on land at ocean beaches. He may then start wondering why people are in the habit of sealing bottles before throwing them into the sea. But he would be mistaken if he tried to draw a conclusion from his findings. There is no general rule compelling people to seal their empty bottles before they are discarded. The simple fact is that only those sealed keep afloat while the others sink to the bottom of the sea with only negligible chances of being seen again by human eyes.

The psychiatrist seeking to sift and classify the evidence for telepathic occurrences which he may come across in his practice must beware of similar false generalizations. Telepathic occurrences that catch his eye are always "striking." Failing this they may easily pass unnoticed. Yet they must not be mistaken for representative samples of the real thing. To put it in technical terms: there is a tendency to consider only those incidents that show unmistakable tracer effects as scientific proof upon which the discussion of telepathic phenomena can be based. But I have pointed out that incidents of this kind are few and far between and in any case atypical. Telepathy is rarely "tagged" with unequivocal identification marks to help the investigators in their appraisal—only few bottles are corked before they are thrown into the sea. The majority sink to the bottom and are never heard of again.

The telepathic dream which is chosen as the point of departure of our argument is of the nature of the sealed bottle washed ashore by the ocean. As such it remains an isolated incident in

* Published in part in the *Amer. J. Psychother.*, IV, 1950.

the case history of the dreamer but it will be seen that she has been subject to recurrent experiences suggestive of telepathy, though of lesser evidential value. Ruth is an unmarried woman of thirty-eight, the youngest of three children. Her mother died while giving birth to Ruth. Her father, a man of commanding personality but old-fashioned Victorian views, never married again. Her mother's sister, an old maid, full of good intentions, moved into the household and was responsible for the girl's upbringing. Her father took to drinking, suffered financial setbacks and grew increasingly morose. He often frightened the child with unexpected outbursts of temper and openly preferred Ruth's sister, Mary, five years her senior, and an older brother. This gave her the feeling that he held her responsible for her mother's death. She found only one effective way to attract her father's attention: she made him laugh with her deliberately silly remarks—with what her family called "Ruth's baby talk." She accepted the role of a dumb-bell, showed little interest in her school work, and was shy and inhibited with boys. In her early teens the meals she shared with her father were a nightmare. She never knew what to say, how to amuse him, how to make him laugh. He, in turn, would embarrass her in front of strangers. He would offer her a quarter for "getting" the meaning of a joke or would tease her by promising money rewards to a boy who would take her out on a date.

On her first date with a young man she felt nauseated. This reaction recurred later whenever she was sexually excited. She felt awkward in company and was unduly concerned over a slight growth of hair on her chest. This was in fact one of her reasons for avoiding intimacies with men. Her father died when she was twenty-three. Three years later she formed an attachment to Henry, a bachelor, twenty-five years older than she. He was a compulsion neurotic and impotent, but appeared to her as the personification of all the masculine virtues she had admired in her father. Her attitude towards him was in many respects a direct continuation of her relationship with the former. He patronized her in a somewhat condescending manner, took her out for dinners, encouraged her baby talk and enjoyed teasing her in a thinly-veiled sadistic fashion, as had her father. At that time she developed vomiting and diarrhoea, increasing anxiety and nightmares of suffocation. Finally she broke off her relationship with Henry and became engaged to a man of her own age. However, this man proved to be a homosexual and, like Henry, impotent. Following this renewed disappointment Ruth developed paranoid ideas. She thought the FBI was after her for falsifying her age in her passport. She felt that people were watching her and saying she was an "old maid." When seeing a gangster picture in the cinema she felt she might be accused of the crime.

Her analysis soon revealed a marked fixation on her father. In her behaviour towards the therapist she sought to repeat the old pattern: she was anxious to please, and tried her best to entertain me with her chatter during the treatment sessions. Her positive transference was unmistakable and ushered in a symptomatic improvement of her condition. At that time, on March 10, 1948, she produced the following dream:

"I went to my dressmaker's with Henry's sister Anne. The dressmaker showed me her place and said the apartment was to let. We looked at it. It consisted of a beautiful long, well-shaped living room, spacious, with high ceiling. It opened out to a nice open terrace where the sun shone. It was long; it stretched along the whole building across the front . . . some 50 feet or so. It had a brick wall and the floor was made of planks with cracks in between. There was not much furniture in the room, not so much as you would have if you would furnish it yourself. There was quite a lot of space left between the things. It was not a cluttered room. There was no carpet, only oriental rugs, a big one in the middle with figures like the one you have here in the office. There were smaller rugs at either end. But they covered only part of the floor, much of it was showing. There were also a few mahogany chairs and an open fireplace. A french door and two french windows opened to the terrace. A dingy little hall led into the bedroom and into a bathroom. I thought this would be the apartment I would like to live in, except that it did not have a maid's room and no extra bathroom. Still, I was wondering how that little dressmaker could afford such a nice apartment. . . ."

The patient's associations shed little light on the deeper

meaning of the dream. She had always considered Anne, Henry's sister, her rival for his affection. Anne was therefore a representative of the patient's own sister, Mary, with whom she had in vain competed for her father's love. Her dressmaker was a somewhat masculine woman whom she nicknamed Bangs on account of her hairdo. She had a tiny apartment on the second floor of an apartment house in Upper Manhattan. She rated her dressmaker either high or rather low in her favours, according to the way she had catered to her sartorial needs. This was the connecting link between Bangs and myself, whom she expected to cater to her psychological needs. The patient had been looking for a new apartment where she could live by herself—not with her tiresome old aunt, as she did at present. Here ended her chain of associations. They revealed nothing about the reason for the appearance in the dream of the detailed picture of the apartment, its precise layout and furnishings, and still less about its relevance to the patient's problems.

But we shall presently see that more light can be thrown on the dream by considering the psychological situation on my side of the picture. A week before the dream occurred, on March 3rd, I had moved into a new apartment in a residential suburb of New York. It was in a large unfinished apartment house and I had been glad to settle down in it comfortably after nearly ten years of nomadic existence during the war. On the night of the dream my brother and his wife had arrived from the country to visit us for the first time in our new home. They shared my enthusiasm. It was a dark rainy night but we stepped out on the terrace which belonged to the apartment. A french door and two french windows opened to the terrace from the living room. It ran across the whole building from one end to the other—between two street blocks—though only a stretch of about 50 by 22 feet was our own. The living room extending into the hall was spacious and high, 34 by 12 feet. It was only scantily furnished at the time the dream occurred. It contained bookshelves on one side; a settee, three easy chairs, two end tables and a small coffee table. On the other end, in the hall, there was only a studio couch and a large unpainted wooden chest. There was no carpet in the apartment, but the floor of the living room was covered by one larger and two smaller oriental rugs, leaving much of the wooden floor uncovered. These rugs were of the same type as I had in my office. A small "dingy" hall led from the living room to the bedroom. It also opened to the bathroom and a second bedroom, occupied by my daughter. The furniture was modern, functional, bleached walnut. There were no mahogany chairs, no fireplace. The main entrance was not from the dingy hall but from the staircase into the hall-living room. The apartment and terrace were on the second floor. The terrace formed the ceiling of the garages belonging to the house. It had a brick wall. At the time the dream occurred the wooden casing of its cemented roof had not yet been removed. It was unfinished and covered with a layer of tarred paper. At one place there was a gaping hole in the floor.

I have to add here that the dreamer located the apartment she saw on the second floor. She made a drawing of its layout as reproduced here.

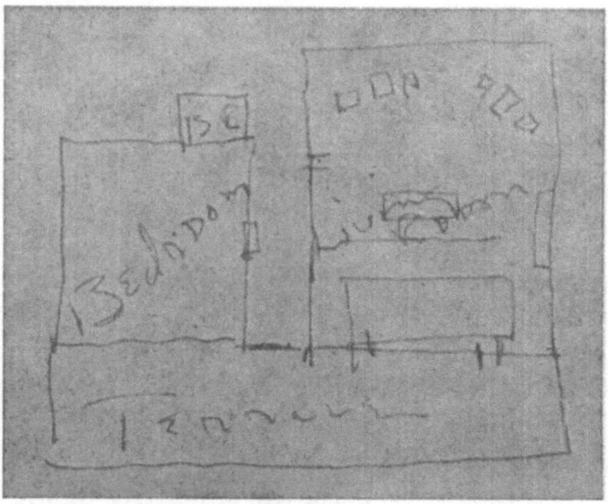

FIG. 1.—Ruth's sketch of her "dream apartment."

It will be noted that her sketch suggests an apartment in a small house, some 50 feet long ("the terrace runs from one end of the house to the other, some 50 feet long"). This is at variance with the fact that both my own and the dressmaker's

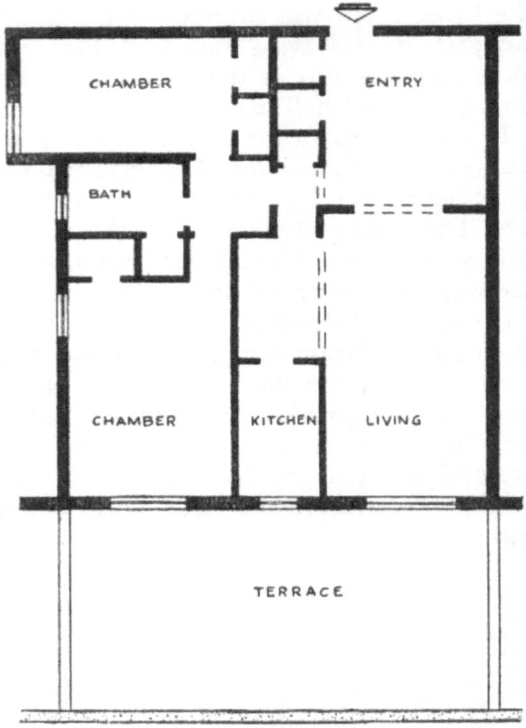

FIG. 2.—Floor plan of the therapist's apartment.

apartments are in large apartment houses. On the other hand, the fact is that Ruth had lived as a child with her father in a self-contained house of the Colonial type. The mahogany furniture seen in her dream was the same, she said, as they had at home. The fireplace, too, reminded her of their sitting room in X. There was no terrace.

In spite of these differences, the similarity of the apartment seen by the patient in her dream and my own apartment is striking enough. The majority of the elements mentioned are independent features of whatever apartment they may belong to, although it may be stated that some are inter-related (several rugs—the floor showing in between; location of bedroom and bathroom, etc.). On the other hand, the whole layout of the place, the references to the large terrace with the parapet running across the house, with the french door and windows opening into it; the oriental rugs, etc., are so specific that the correspondences cannot reasonably be attributed to chance alone. Indeed, the chance hypothesis would explain nothing in our case. On the contrary, it would rather bar the way for a proper understanding even of the familiar psychoanalytic aspects of the dream.

The corresponding features can be listed in the table below:

Dream	*Reality*
(1) Spacious high living room.	(1) Spacious high living room.
(2) French door and windows to terrace.	(2) French door and windows to terrace.
(3) Very large terrace running across the house.	(3) Very large terrace running across the house.
(4) Brick parapet on terrace.	(4) Brick parapet on terrace.
(5) Scanty furniture in living room "not as you would furnish it yourself."	(5) Scanty furniture in living room (European taste).
(6) Oriental rugs "like here in the office."	(6) Oriental rugs of the identical type.
(7) One large rug, two smaller ones on both sides.	(7) One large rug, two smaller ones on both sides.
(8) Leaving floor uncovered in places.	(8) Leaving floor uncovered in places.
(9) Bedroom located to the east of living room.	(9) Bedroom located to the east of living room.
(10) Bathroom located to the east of living room.	(10) Bathroom located to the east of living room.
(11) Dingy little hall connecting (9) and (10) with living room.	(11) "Dingy" little hall connecting (9) and (10) with living room.
(12) No maid's room.	(12) No maid's room.
(13) No second bathroom.	(13) No second bathroom.

For the sake of the records I have to add here that the patient had been completely ignorant of my personal circumstances before and during the whole course of the treatment. She did not know my private address or telephone number, she had been unaware of my moving to a new apartment and could by no conceivable "normal" ways of communication have learned about its size, layout and furnishings.

I mentioned, however, that there is also a number of points of difference between the dream and reality. I may only recall the mahogany chairs and the fireplace which reminded her of her father's apartment. This indicates that the apartment seen in the dream represents something like a composite picture of her own childhood home and my residence. It is a product of the dream work in which what I described as autopsychic material, derived from early recollections, is condensed with heteropsychic material of telepathic origin.

This interpretation accounts for both the correspondences and divergencies found in the manifest dream content as compared with its two sources: autopsychic and heteropsychic. It is in this way—and in this way only—that we can arrive at a better understanding of the dream. I hinted that the patient's associations left a major part of its manifest content unaccounted for. But once we realize the origin of that material from outside, that is, from a heteropsychic source, we are able to close the gap. More than that: we arrive at a better understanding of the patient's attitude towards myself and towards the treatment at the time the dream occurred. It quite obviously dramatizes her wish to move into my apartment and to live there with me as she did with her father during her childhood years. It expresses Ruth's positive transference upon the therapist. The presence of Anne, the sister of the man to whom she had clung for many years as to another father substitute, completes the picture. Anne is the replica of her own sister Mary, who had usurped her place in her father's affection. Now the apartment with the large terrace and the fireplace was to become hers, and Anne, the rival, is just an onlooker. By taking sole possession of her dream house, one of her cherished childhood dreams had indeed come true.

At this point I should like to insert a few remarks about the psychological setting on "my end" at the time of Ruth's dream. I mentioned that it coincided with my brother's arrival from the country. Yet, as it happened, seeing my new home was not the sole purpose of his coming. We had just learned from our mother in England that she had suddenly been taken ill and that an operation had become necessary. We had therefore good reason to try to hasten her coming to this country—a project that met with considerable difficulties. We had also agreed that on her arrival here she should live in my new home until better arrangements could be made for her permanent accommodation. This plan touched on the problem of where my daughter, aged thirteen, would live on my mother's arrival; on my concern over the way in which relationships in our extended little family group were to work out, and on a host of other rather personal problems which need not be discussed here in greater detail.

It would be tempting to go into more details of my own reaction to—or counter-transference on—my patient. Be it sufficient to note that I felt somewhat threatened by her growing dependence on me and ill at ease as the sole recipient of her filial devotion. Yet at the same time I did not want to discourage her positive transference by premature interpretations and I felt I had to maintain my role as a protective father figure in the interest of the treatment. To what extent playing such a role also met certain personality needs of my own is another question. I may only point to my concern over my daughter's privacy, the eventual need to exile her from her room on my mother's arrival. In retrospect all these points appear of a trivial nature. But they throw light on the special relevance of Ruth's dream to my own problems at the time her dream occurred and give deeper insight into its dynamics. Ruth expressed her positive transference to me in a series of dreams recorded some time before. One dream was as follows: "You were annoyed with me because I don't try hard enough. I was afraid you would drop me and say I have to stop and that my further coming would be just a waste of time and money."

The dream obviously expressed her need for encouragement and affection which she thought she would receive by stressing her submissive attitude towards me. In another dream she saw me dressed in a lugubrious black suit. I reprimanded her for her behaviour like a stern forbidding person. The black suit reminded her of the one that Henry, her bachelor friend, used to wear. The stern forbidding person was her father.

A week or so later she related a dream about Henry, who was away on a trip to Europe.

"Henry died from heart attack in Italy. I had just had lunch with somebody at the beach . . . perhaps it was Tom, my new boy friend. I saw Henry lying dead on a table. I felt his face. It was not cold at all. I kissed his cheek but he did not open his eyes. I was not grieved, but I felt part of my inside dead."

It is not necessary to go into all the unconscious implications of this dream. On a superficial level it shows her ambivalent feelings towards Henry, her father surrogate, her love and hatred towards him. It also shows her on the point of breaking away from him and of replacing him by Tom. Although inclined to be superstitious, Ruth was not disturbed by this dream. She admitted that Henry was no longer an integral part of her life and that she had severed the ties which had existed between them. Henry dead or alive—she was free to live on without him. Tom was a man a few years younger than Ruth. She had formed a sexual attachment to him and had become increasingly involved in the new relationship. At the same time her gastro-intestinal symptoms subsided: she no longer felt sick when sexually excited. She had also overcome her fear of being regarded as a Lesbian, of being watched by people, and other symptoms of her paranoid trend.

It will be noted from this account that apart from the telepathic dream recorded here there have been no further instances of telepathy in Ruth's case history. The dream about Henry's death contained no telepathic elements. As far as can be said without information about the psychological situation on his side, it was derived from purely autopsychic sources. Henry returned home from abroad safe and well, the same old eccentric he had been before.

There are, however, indications that Ruth had on several previous occasions experiences of a similar nature, though of lesser evidential value. This is illustrated by the following example. One night she dreamed that she was falling from an airplane from the height of 27,000 feet. Her free associations led her to Jules Verne's book, *Twenty Thousand Leagues Under the Sea*; to the fear of water and the fear of drowning. While listening to the chain of her associations I suddenly got the impression, "This is how she must have responded to the Rorschach test she was given by Dr. Harrower three or four months ago." At that moment the patient adds: "And that reminds me of choking, of that *harrowble* . . . horrible feeling of choking, and that Dr. Harrower asked me 'What are you most afraid of' and I said 'of drowning'." This would indicate that her slip of the tongue was due to telepathy from myself to the patient. But we cannot rule out two other possible explanations. It could be stated that the associations of both Ruth and myself were conditioned by what we knew about Dr. Harrower's method of testing. Yet, I have to add here that I found no indications in Dr. Harrower's notes that the question quoted by Ruth had been part of the examination, nor did I know that it was one of the stock questions put by the clinical psychologist to his subject. I had therefore no apparent reason to think of Dr. Harrower before the patient made the slip. If this is true my own trend of thought ("This is how she must have responded to the psychological test") would be due to telepathy in the reverse direction: from the patient to the analyst.

Another incident was reported to me by Ruth herself. One day she was involved in a conversation about a topic which she knew to be far beyond her. Two friends discussed the question of how much the city of M. would spend on education in a year. "Two hundred thousand dollars" she remarked in a casual way. Right or wrong, this was exactly the figure her friend had in mind. Ruth had of course not the slightest notion about the city's budget, educational or otherwise, nor about her friend's estimate of it.

It is true that this incident is of even more doubtful evidential value than the telepathic nature of the slip of her tongue. Moreover, it rests entirely with the patient's own authority. However, there are other instances in which I gained the impression that Ruth did indeed possess an unusual ability to "sense" the mental or emotional state of other people. One day she met Miss Z. in my waiting room. Miss Z. had passed through a severe emotional crisis during the preceding session. Ruth could not have caught more than a brief glance of the patient, but she had grasped the situation in a flash and expressed her concern over Miss Z. in a way which only confirmed my own impression. At a later session she met the same patient again for a brief moment and was greatly relieved by the progress she could see. Her observation again hit the nail on the head.

There is another side of her behaviour which illustrates the same point. From the beginning of her analysis Ruth was eager to accommodate herself to the limits of her capacities to what she thought was my own scale of values and philosophy of life. She expressed the desire to complete her college education, to take up painting or modelling, or to open, at least, a book shop of her own in order to cease being what she called a social parasite and to become a useful member of the community. She bought books on subjects far beyond her depth and sought to involve me in discussions about learned matters. The following dream illustrates this phase.

"I went with my former fiancé into a panelled library. He pulled a book out of the shelf; it was *Aeneas* by Virgil in 'blank verse.' I thought he was smart. But when he put his arm around me I thought how silly of him to think that this means something to me."

When I yielded to the temptation to encourage her intellectual ambitions, she became irritable and anxious again. Yet all her new symptoms subsided rapidly when I hinted that there was no need to go out of her way in order to please me in the manner she had tried to please her father and that she might just as well continue to live her own life.

From the psychoanalytic point of view there can be little doubt that all these vicissitudes of Ruth's response to the treatment have to be attributed to two chief causes: to unconscious suggestive elements contained in my approach to the patient, and to fluctuations of her transference on the therapist. The fact is that easy suggestibility had been one of her outstanding features. Since early childhood she had been in the habit of having her thoughts, judgments, and predilections directed by others. It is readily understood that the psychoanalytic situation, despite its primary rational objective, made her all the more susceptible to influences of this kind. Like many hysterics and some borderline schizophrenics Ruth herself had developed a technique of her own in using her sensitiveness to her best advantage. She kept a watchful eye on the moods and personal idiosyncrasies of those around her, eager to respond to the slightest clue she could cull from their demeanour. She was hypersensitive to the subtlest signs of approval or disapproval, particularly by those whom she tended to identify with her father.

All this resulted in increasing the keenness of her observation—conscious or unconscious—and in the gradual development of what in common parlance would be called her intuitive abilities. It is obviously impossible to decide whether and how far here, too, a telepathic factor is involved. I pointed out in the introductory remarks that even though we may be able to offer a clear-cut conceptual definition of the telepathic process we must not expect to find telepathy in everyday life without an admixture of sensory perception. More often than not telepathy may be indistinguishable from the give and take of the familiar means of human intercommunication. Words spoken and unspoken may assume a deeper meaning by subtle inflections or intonations of voice, by unconscious expressive movements—and their unconscious appreciation—without telepathy being involved in the process. Conversely, it may well be that minute sensory clues given away by the analyst (and usually regarded as vehicles of unintended suggestion) at the same time contain a telepathic component.

It would be futile, therefore, to ask how much of the suggestive element that can be found in the analytic situation is of telepathic nature, and how much of the alleged telepathic effects should more conveniently be explained by suggestion. The two processes are not mutually exclusive. They may go hand in hand and reinforce each other. They are obviously not a matter of either-or, but of both-the-one-and-the-other.

It is the difficulty of drawing a strict demarcation line between unmistakably telepathic elements on the one hand and between subliminal sensory clues (or what McCleary and Lazarus[79] have described as *sub-ceptions*) on the other, which is one of the major obstacles in coming to grips with our problem.

In the case of Ruth's apartment dream at least the objection of subliminal sensory clues can be ruled out of the question. It is therefore a good example of an incident whose supposed telepathic nature is suggested by the combination of two criteria which were discussed in the preceding chapter: (1) both the manifest dream content and the therapist's emotionally charged thoughts and preoccupations at the time of the dream contain a variety of specific distinctive features whose close correspondence cannot reasonably be attributed to chance alone; (2) the telepathic interpretation of the dream is supported by the criterion of psychological significance or consistency of such an interpretation. Indeed, I indicated that it is only through such an interpretation that we can close the gap in our understanding of the latent meaning of the dream and reach a deeper insight into its dynamics. Failing this a large portion of the dream remains unintelligible.

CHAPTER IV

Ronald's Telepathic Dream

THE telepathic dream reported by our next patient throws more light upon the psychodynamics of the telepathic process. At the same time it confronts the therapist with a new and somewhat disconcerting situation: it shows that, despite the attitude of detachment and reserve which he seeks to maintain during the treatment, he may become more involved with his patient's problems than is allowed for by psychoanalytic theory, and that, on a deeper level, his patients may themselves have a far greater awareness of his involvement than may ever occur to the analyst. We shall see on a later page that this unconscious involvement of the therapist constitutes a new challenge to his analytical self-searching. Indeed, it places the responsibility upon him of paying unremitting attention to both aspects of the psychoanalytic situation: to that represented by the patient's own—autopsychic—productions as well as to that which is revealed by the patient's occasional telepathic responses to the therapist's unconscious. This is what I described as the method of comparative analysis.[32] It involves constant scrutiny of the therapist's counter-transference and is indispensable for the dynamic understanding of telepathy both inside and outside the analytic situation.

The dream reported by Ronald H., a war veteran of twenty-five, studying under the GI Bill, is as follows: "I am with my sister or with my wife in a house beside a stream. A flight of stairs leads up to the house. The stairs go round the corner up to a landing. There is a little green field on one side of the house. The sun shines on it; it is beautiful. I understand it belongs to Warner Brothers and I am not supposed to go there. It is lower than the house. The house is luxurious, attractive, made in part of greyish black stone. A wall of greyish black rocks surrounds the little field on the right side of the house. There is a hill in the background."

Ronald has been my patient during the ten preceding months. He is suffering from a compulsion neurosis with marked emotional blocking and perfectionistic tendencies. He is the youngest of three brothers and has been exposed to much bullying by them. A younger sister is aged twenty-four. His father was a strict disciplinarian who kept him in constant fear of his temperamental outbursts. He describes his mother as the victim of his father's brutal temper, and when the patient was twelve years of age she suffered a nervous breakdown and had to be admitted to a mental hospital.

At the age of thirteen one of Ronald's older brothers forced him to engage in sex play. There are two more instances of homosexual seduction in his case history.

Like many compulsion neurotics the patient had much intellectual insight into his difficulties. He was himself able to offer a partial interpretation of his dream. The sunny, green field, he stated, represented temptation. The prohibition to go there meant the denial of giving in to temptation. It was on a "lower level" to which he was not allowed to descend. This he associated with his incestuous feelings towards his sister who was to be engaged soon and who therefore had become still more inaccessible to him than ever before.

To *Warner* Brothers he associated a *warning* to the brothers to behave themselves and to refrain from homosexual activities or incest. The warning, he felt, came from his father.

He had no association to account for the stream. It should be noted that when sketching the scene in which the dream took place he first drew one line only, omitting the other bank of the river (Fig. 3). The line representing the other bank he inserted only after the therapist had drawn his attention to its omission. In this way the original drawing indicated a lake rather than a stream.

Neither was the patient able to offer any association in connection with the house. The wall or the rocks surrounding the grassy patch reminded him of the scenery close to the hospital to which his mother had been admitted. It may well be that at this point we have to resort to the symbolic interpretation of both house and stream (or lake) in terms of the human body. They may be taken to represent his mother,

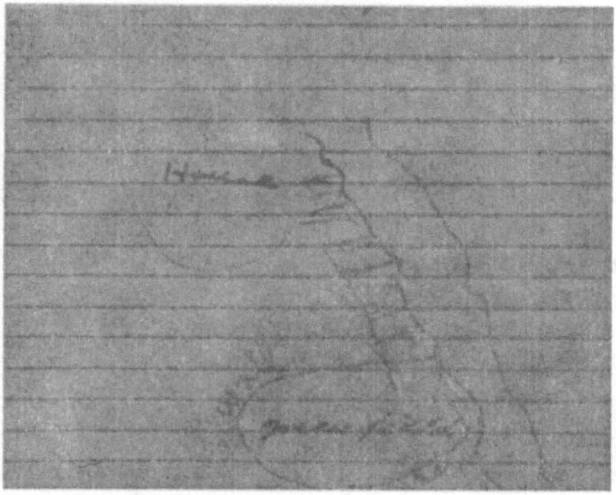

FIG. 3.—Ronald's Dream.

indicating his desire to return to her—i.e. for a symbolic reunion with his sister and brothers in the maternal womb. On another level this desire may be related to suppressed anal tendencies which are known to play an important part in the character structure of patients of his type.

Here, again, more light can be thrown on the psychodynamics of the dream by considering the psychological situation on my side of the picture. The patient had the dream on a Sunday night in the early spring of 1950. As it happened I had made a trip to the countryside on the same Sunday in search of a summer house which my family and I planned to share with friends. It was a beautiful spring day and the house offered to me by the real estate agent exceeded all my expectations. It was situated on the shore of a lake, perched between shrubbery and rock formations. A wooden staircase led up to a spacious porch. A small pier was situated on the left of the house. On the right side, sloping toward the lake, there was a small grassy beach, illuminated by the afternoon sun. It was the only spot in the immediate vicinity of the house holding the promise of peaceful relaxation on the lake front. It was surrounded by greyish black rock formations, characteristic of the whole district. The house was richly furnished as summer houses go. In any case, it seemed luxurious when compared with the cottages I had occupied in preceding summers. Notwithstanding the fairly high rent asked by the agent both I and members of my family were enthusiastic about the place. Moreover, our friends had already inspected the house on the preceding Sunday and made tentative arrangements for renting it. They had also given the agent a considerable deposit. Only a few formalities remained to be settled between the present writer and the owner of the property when the conversation turned to the grassy patch at the right of the house. This patch, Mr. S. remarked, was not to be used by the tenants. It belonged to other houses a quarter of a mile away and was out of bounds for us. He brushed aside our objections by remarking that the small pier on the left would well serve our purpose. He warned us at the same time that he would object to any overcrowding of the house whose sanitary facilities could cater only for a limited number of occupants. Mr. S. was a tough American business man and I have to admit that I felt in no position to argue my point with such an opponent. I left with the feeling that I would have to take the place despite the strings attached to the lease.

On discussing the matter with our friends on the same evening it was decided, however, that Mr. S.'s new terms were unacceptable and that to our regret we had to reverse our original decision. Unfortunately Mr. S. proved to be even tougher than he had first appeared. Not only was he unwilling to make any concessions but he also refused to return the deposit. Thus what might have been the prelude to a pleasant summer vacation ended with a note of jarring discord and disappointment for all concerned.

What, then, is the relevance of these strictly personal matters to the dream dreamt by our patient?

On examining the events that had happened on my end on the day of the dream in greater detail, a certain correspondence between a number of distinctive features in the manifest content of the dream and in reality is unmistakable. There is, first, the mention of a "luxurious" house on the water front. There are, secondly, the greyish black rock formations in its vicinity. There is, thirdly, an outdoor staircase leading up to it;

there is, fourth, a beautiful grassy patch on the lower level at its right. There is, further, a *warning* that just this desirable spot is out of bounds to both the patient and the therapist and, lastly, there is the fact that a warning comes from a frustrating parental figure in the one case, and from a person evoking old memories of similar conflicts with a punitive father figure in the other. We find in this way a multiplicity of distinctive features common to two contemporaneous sets of mental events whose coincidence it would be difficult to attribute to chance alone.

Still, the question remained whether or not the chance explanation could entirely be ruled out of the question. In order to make at least one step towards clarifying this point a simple experiment was carried out, using the sketch made by the patient and nine control drawings prepared by the present writer. The control drawings, made on the same type of paper and similar in style to the one sketched by the patient, represented a random collection of crude street maps, e.g. a map of the area of Central Park; of a train entering a tunnel; of an airship passing through clouds, etc.

The ten drawings were shown to:

1. the writer's wife, 2. his daughter,
3. Mr. N., 4. Mrs. N.,
5. Mr. U., 6. Mrs. U.,

all of whom had shared with the present writer the lakeside experience as described above, although on different days.

The showing of the pictures was accompanied by a few explanatory remarks, e.g. "Here is a train going into a tunnel"; or "Here is a grassy patch to the right of the house to which no one is admitted." The subjects were asked individually and independently of each other to say what specific scene or experience they were reminded of by the drawings. The first four subjects questioned in this way identified Ronald's "dream house" without hesitation as the one seen on the lakeside a week or so ago. The remaining two, Mr. and Mrs. U., were shown the drawings after a six weeks' interval. The drawing failed to make any impression on them and did not recall the faded memory of the lakeside incident.

Many objections can be raised to this experiment, e.g. as regards the mathematics involved, the inadequate randomization of the control drawings, and the failure to show the same drawings to controls not involved in the experience. However, it should be noted here that the nature of the material contained in the dream is by itself prohibitive to strictly mathematical treatment. For the same reason any attempt at more stringent randomization of the control drawings seemed to be unnecessary. More relevant is the objection that the instructions given by the experimenter might have included clues apt to give the "game" away, regardless of the presence or absence of any tell-tale resemblances in the drawing itself. It can be objected that the very mention of the sunlit grassy patch to which access is denied to the dreamer might have conveyed a hint as to what the experimenter had in mind—particularly in view of the experience so recently shared by both himself and his companions. But it goes without saying that in omitting this clue from his instructions the experimenter would have failed to convey to his subjects one of the principal features of the dream. In fact, it was the reference to the "prohibited area" in the dream which contained the key word for its first tentative identification by the present writer as presumptively telepathic.

I must stress the fact that the test with the four subjects whose responses amounted to a positive identification was carried out within a week after the incident described. The two remaining subjects were tested six weeks later—with negative result. Both the drawings and the experimenter's instructions failed to strike responsive chords. Obviously, in Mr. and Mrs. U. the common experience had already lost its recency and thereby its psychological significance.

If this is true the objection that the experimenter's explanatory remarks had given the game away is no longer tenable. We have to realize that if it is right to consider his reference to the prohibited grassy patch as a tell-tale clue of sufficient significance it is only fair to grant that his own response to the patient's account of his dream amounted largely to the same thing as the reaction of his four "positive" subjects. The difference between the two responses lies only in the fact that, while his subjects had shared with him the knowledge of an actual incident, the patient could have received the same information only in a telepathic way.

It may be well to revert at this point to the psychodynamic aspects of our case. I hinted that on seeking to evaluate the psychological significance of a particular *motif* or element contained in the manifest content of a dream, it is not enough to confine ourselves to making an inventory of a few more or less conspicuous elements whose presumable telepathic correspondence with a real event is then discussed in terms of probability, calculable or otherwise. We have to determine the specific weight, as it were, of the element concerned and to decide on its merits whether or not its telepathic interpretation meets the criterion of psychological significance.

I mentioned that in the dream considered here the *motif* of banishment and denial—"You must not trespass on this ground"—had emerged as its principal feature. As far as the dreamer was concerned this warning referred to his unconscious incestuous wishes directed towards his sister and mother and, on a deeper level, perhaps to repressed anal tendencies. I also indicated that my own frustrating lakeside experience hit upon similar repressed problems of my own. Much in the same way as my patient, I too was unduly taken aback by Mr. S.'s injunction, and, on analysis of my failure to take a more aggressive stand against him, it would be easy to demonstrate the close resemblance of what was left of my Oedipal—and perhaps pregenital—conflicts with the corresponding conflicts of my patient. If this is true, it could be stated that it is at the exact intersection of the emotional trends represented by our respective conflicts that the described telepathic incident had taken place. It is as though the patient had sensed the therapist's vulnerability on this score, telling him: "You too are struggling with the same problem as I. You too are a *brother* who is *warned* by a threatening parental figure to keep out of trouble. In fact, you have not fared much better in resolving your conflict with your father than I have."

It is true that on reducing the latent meaning of the dream and of my emotional reaction to the forbidding Mr. S. to this ultimate core we have descended to a level on which in all probability all men, women, and children reared in our culture would reveal basic similarities of their repressed instinctual drives. The Oedipus conflict and certain pregenital taboos and guilt feelings have become common characteristics of modern man's personality structure and their presence in both therapist and patient certainly cannot be invoked as evidence of something like telepathic correspondence between them.

Yet it should be recalled at this point that it is not the duplication of this universal pattern of conflict, common perhaps to all mankind, but the correspondence of a particular set of clearly identifiable distinctive features in dream and reality upon which, in our argument, the claim of telepathy is based. In fact, I pointed out on an earlier page that only such tracer effects as are provided by the presence of specific distinctive features in the manifest content of a dream should be regarded as stringent criteria of telepathy in a concrete case.

This disposes at the same time of an important objection Paul Schilder[110] has made as long as twenty years ago to the psychoanalytic treatment of the problems of telepathy. Schilder warned that the very presence of such universal archetypal patterns as can be found at the roots of dreams and other manifestations of the unconscious might easily be mistaken as proofs of telepathic correspondences. We will see in Chapter XVI that Schilder's argument might be advanced also in the reverse direction. It might be stated that the universality of certain archetypal images in our mental make-up is itself due to a basic process of sharing which is barely distinguishable from what is commonly described as telepathy and that it is only the absence of telepathic tracer effects which makes the telepathic interpretation of their universal occurrence a matter of conjecture rather than of scientific proof. (Whoever is inclined to raise objection to such an interpretation should not overlook that the occurrence of archetypal patterns is itself merely a more or less empirical fact unaccounted for so far in terms of a valid scientific explanatory hypothesis.)

Nevertheless, the presence of two corresponding and structurally analogous complexes in both agent and percipient does not by itself suffice to account for the telepathic incidents described. If this were the case we should come across a much greater number of telepathic incidents in our daily practice than actually come to our notice. Obviously a multiplicity of other factors have to be present for that purpose.

Here, too, more can be learned by closer inquiry into the transference relationship between therapist and patient at the time the dream occurred. Analysis revealed that the patient had assumed much the same submissive, feminine attitude towards the therapist as he had shown in his relationship to his father. The passive homosexual colouring of this attitude had become increasingly obvious and was expressed in his free associations. I have to remark at this point that in this attitude, he was under the direct influence of Fred L., another patient of mine, with whom he had been on friendly terms and whose neurosis showed certain resemblances to his own. Moreover, Fred had been much less reticent regarding details of his analysis than was desirable from the therapeutic point of view. It was as though Ronald had been competing with Fred, his senior colleague, in whatever analytic progress he had made, saying: "If you can dig up such and such early infantile material from your unconscious—so can I!"

In fact, Ronald was fully aware of his competitive attitude with his friend and brother-in-arms and repeatedly commented on it. There is, however, another aspect of their competitive relationship which had escaped his attention at that time. Exactly a year prior to the telepathic dream discussed here, Fred had been involved in a series of telepathic incidents during analysis which will be described in the next chapter. Fred had become cognizant of these occurrences and there is reason to believe that he had mentioned them to his junior colleague. This may in turn have sparked the latter's desire to emulate the accomplishments of his friend. It is as though he said in his dream: "Not only can I produce the same kind of repressed material from my unconscious [i.e. from the autopsychic sphere] as Fred, I can also outdo him so far as telepathy is concerned. I can supply heteropsychic material which, I am sure, will please my analyst just as much as whatever my rival could offer."

It has to be admitted here that Ronald was not altogether mistaken in this respect. I have to confess that at certain stages of my analytical work I have not been entirely able to dispel a sense of expectancy regarding the possible occurrence of telepathic incidents. But it may also be fair to say that in this respect my position is not altogether different from that of my more orthodox colleagues. They too cannot help approaching their task with certain tacit assumptions and expectations which are then put to the test of the patient's reaction in the psychoanalytic situation. Early writings of Freud[44c] himself contain many references to that effect. The fact that scientific expectations of this kind, derived in part from past experience and in part from analytic training and indoctrination, may indeed influence the material obtained in the analytic situation itself will be discussed in the chapter dealing with the problem of telepathic leakage.

If this is true, it is readily understood that by the same token the very expectancy on the part of the therapist of telepathic occurrences may well serve as an added predisposing factor for their occurrence—provided that such other factors as the patient's readiness to answer his call meet halfway his own personality needs.

Our observation that telepathy may occur on the exact point of intersection of two corresponding or converging emotional trends in patient and therapist is thus to be supplemented by the statement that its emergence may be further aided by the emotionally charged interest of those involved in the subject-matter of telepathic communication itself and by their desire to establish such a communication.

CHAPTER V

More Telepathic Incidents During Analysis

*The Case of Fred L.**

THE case history of our next patient contains more observations suggestive of telepathy in the psychoanalytic situation. Some of the incidents closely follow the pattern of the dreams discussed in the previous chapters. Others, again, are less revealing from the psychoanalytic point of view and therefore less significant for a study chiefly concerned with the dynamics of such incidents. This should not, however, justify their omission in the present context.

Brushing aside material of this kind would only lead to a one-sided picture of the telepathic process. We have to realize that the study of *psi* functions—like the study of psychology in general—has to be based on a combined phenomenological and dynamic approach. It has to admit all the data that come to its notice, however trifling and inconsequential they may appear. It will be seen, moreover, that in addition to a number of more or less trivial incidents, the same patient produced two telepathic dreams which readily lend themselves to psychoanalytic exploration.

Fred L. is a close friend of Ronald, the college student, whose dream was described in the previous chapter. He is two years his senior and had entered analysis about a year before him. Fred has been suffering from an obsessive compulsive neurosis from childhood. From the age of eleven or twelve he has had various sado-masochistic fantasies which stayed with him until the time he commenced treatment at twenty-seven. He had the compulsion to ask his girl friend whether she was

* Published in part in *Psychiatr. Quart.*, 24, 1950.

"stronger" than Mrs. X. or Mrs. Y. He felt the impulse to kick women he saw in the street. He had to count compulsively the number of tiles in the toilet or of bricks on buildings he passed in the street. At the same time he showed the characteristic perfectionist tendencies of the compulsion neurotic.

He was unmarried and greatly devoted to his mother who, he said, advised him against marrying a divorced woman with whom he had an affair. He was erectively potent but had to resort to his fantasies during intercourse. In analysis he produced a wealth of thinly disguised incestuous material. He dreamt that he had "done wrong"; that the police were after him and that he had taken refuge in his mother's house. In another dream he was struggling with three rattlesnakes, with the scene shifting to a big blustering man who was beating up men and women in a train. The patient did not dare to resist him. The snake *motif* returned in many subsequent dreams. In one he wanted to capture a snake hidden in the grass. He was barefoot and felt it was too dangerous to try. He blamed his father who did not buy him shoes. In the same dream he saw a huge fat fish, three times his own size, lying next to the snake. The fish reminded him of his mother.

Despite the obvious meaning of most of the material produced during the initial stage of the treatment, no interpretations were given to the patient. Analysis was largely confined to his ego-defences, to his ambivalent attitude toward his father and its re-enactment in the transference relationship.

Boxing and wrestling had been Fred's hobbies up to the age of fourteen. At that time he decided to give them up because the thought of hitting people had become revolting to him. He had been a rough and boisterous youngster, member of a tough street gang, given to cruel pranks. He recalls an incident when, while wrestling with a friend, he suddenly stopped hitting him because he was overcome by scruples. From then onward his interest in boxing and wrestling was only theoretical. He daydreamed of showing off his muscles but refrained from any active participation in competitive sports. Withdrawing from the street gang, he became a voracious reader and increasingly interested in abstract philosophical problems. When he began analysis he had already read a great deal of analytical literature.

In contrast to his powerful physical build, he was meek and submissive in his demeanour and overpolite toward the therapist. He would never contradict or protest against a change of appointment and it took him several months until he was capable of expressing hostile feelings.

He was greatly relieved on recognizing these attitudes as reaction formations to his repressed aggressive tendencies. He remembered that as a child of two or three, while horse-playing with his father, he urinated on his head. More memories of this kind followed, mobilizing the patient's castration fears.

Dream: "I broke my upper jaw when I played football or baseball. Some man was to set it. I insisted it should be Dr. C. or Dr. G. but they were too busy. I could not find anybody to do it. It got worse and worse and so I had to pull my front teeth."

He now gave free vent to his hostility against his father, in whose jewellery business he worked as a junior partner. It was expressed in terms of profuse oral and anal sadistic material to which he responded with more and more undisguised castration fantasies. After a transient phase of increased anxiety, during which he lost his potency, his condition showed a marked improvement. Fred had no longer to resort to his sadistic fantasies during intercourse and his potency was restored. At about that time he decided that he would end the partnership with his father and go into business on his own.

In view of this progress I hinted that his treatment might be terminated sooner than expected without, however, specifying the date of termination. As a result of my casual remark the patient passed into a new phase of resistance, accompanied by a new flow of sadistic material. At the same time he professed to be overjoyed by the contemplated end of the treatment. Nevertheless, he was still doubtful as to his ability to stand on his own feet. He knew enough about psychoanalytic theory to wonder if he had recalled and worked through sufficient early infantile material to be safe from a relapse. This he tried to do in his usual compulsive way but produced little of analytic interest or true therapeutic value.

It was at this time, in the twelfth month of his treatment,

that I recorded a series of observations of an apparently telepathic nature.

Dream: "A man was fixing our cellar. He made a window for the cellar bathroom to let in light and fresh air. I thought the window would be too large. Then I thought: No, it would rather be too small. Finally I thought it would be all right. I felt I owed the man something for his labours. I thought I would let him have a piece of jewellery at a reduced price so that I could show him my gratitude. But I could not do it because of my father's objections."

The rest of the dream contained another variation on the theme of his resentment of his father and is irrelevant in the present context. The cellar reminded him of his own unconscious, the bathroom of the wealth of anal material produced in the course of the treatment. Letting in fresh air and light, therefore, referred to his analysis. The man who fixed the cellar was myself. He had no associations connected with the size of the window. With reference to the piece of jewellery he complained that his father had never given him a chance to sell watches or jewellery to his friends at reduced prices.

These associations make the meaning of the dream obvious. It expresses his appreciation of the treatment, his wish to show his gratitude to the therapist—although the resentment expressed in the second part of the dream (not reproduced here) also shows the ambivalent nature of his transference.

As usual in a dream suggestive of the involvement of a telepathic factor, more light can be thrown on its latent meaning by paying attention to the psychological situation on "my end" at the time the dream occurred. On listening to Fred's account of the *fresh air* and *light* that were to be let into the cellar I was struck by the close correspondence of his remark with what I had said two days before to the engineer who was to install an air-conditioning unit in my office. I remarked to him that the office was very much like a *cellar* with very little *air* and *light* coming in and that a large unit, therefore, would not be required. I expressed concern, though, that its only *window would be still more reduced in size*, making the room darker than before. The man assured me that this was not the case; on the contrary, the window would look *larger* than before. When the man left, my wife (who works as my secretary in the office) and I laughed at this somewhat insipid piece of sales talk. But I remarked that he obviously referred to the operation of the fan which would bring in more air in winter than could be let in through the partly open window. Since I used artificial light most of the time, the reduction in daylight coming in through the window would not make any difference at all.

I have to add here that the dream occurred on a Thursday night, in the middle of May 1949, and that the unit was to be installed on the day following the Friday session with my patient, i.e. on Saturday. As indicated, my conversation with the air-conditioning man took place on Wednesday.

Needless to say, the prospect of having such a unit installed in my office had given me quite a thrill. Indeed, the thought of it may have occupied my mind during the preceding days to a greater extent than anybody concerned over his professional dignity would like to confess in public.

The *motif* of the *jewellery* leads to another, not less embarrassing trend of thought. My wife had inherited a rather old-fashioned diamond wristwatch and had expressed the wish to have it reset, preferably by the firm with which Fred had been connected. I indicated to her that asking a patient for such a favour was out of the question, but agreed that she might turn to him once the treatment was terminated. My wife had first brought up the matter about three weeks earlier. Two or three days before the dream occurred I told her that Fred was indeed making good progress and that her "dream" about having her watch reset might eventually come true in the not too distant future.

I have to emphasize at this point that neither my wife nor I had made any reference to the matter in front of the patient, nor had he any inkling of the proposed installation of an air-conditioner in my office. This is important to bear in mind since in the session preceding the one in which he had related the dream he had made another—this time open—reference to an air-conditioner quite "out of the blue."

At that period of the treatment he was in the habit of starting the session with a long string of trivial associations referring to objects seen in the room, to my wife's appearance, etc., interspersed with the monotonous recital of his obsessive-compulsive fantasies. It was in this chain of seemingly incoherent associations that he suddenly referred to a small electric heater (which he had become sufficiently familiar with in the course of the preceding months) as an *air-conditioner.* I recorded his slip without commenting to him on what to me had already on that first occasion appeared as a curious coincidence with my own preconscious preoccupation.

In the fourth session following the incident just described, the patient produced what appears to be another telepathic reaction. Starting his chain of associations in his usual manner he said among other things: "Dirty chair . . . kicking you . . . your wife has golden teeth. . . . She has new shoes today . . . when will this end?", etc. At first, I paid no attention to his remark about my wife's new shoes. Yet, after Fred left I asked her about them. She was surprised. She did buy herself a pair of shoes on her way to the office, before 2 p.m. She did not wear them, nor even unpack them, but put the box down in a small treatment room not directly connected with the office, out of the patient's sight, and indeed, inaccessible to him. The patient had his session at 3 p.m. He had neither seen my wife on her way to the office nor had he encountered her accidentally while she was shopping. I, for my part, had also been unaware of what happened. Nor had I been previously informed of her intention to buy new shoes. In this way, unless we choose to attribute the patient's reaction to the familar *deus ex machina* called chance it may again well be attributable to telepathy—this time from my wife to the patient. It will be noted that the same consideration can be applied both to the air-conditioner and the watch *motifs* that were involved in the previous instances.

The possibility of a joint telepathic agency involving myself as well as my wife is also to be considered in the following incident. The patient described a dream in which he was told by a doctor that he was suffering from anaemia. This set into motion a chain of associations part of which runs as follows: "Anaemia . . . only sissies have anaemia . . . blood . . . blushing. . . . Oilcloth . . . why do I think of oilcloth? . . . is it psychic again? . . . oilcloth in cellar . . . dogs' faeces . . . my girl friend is stronger than your wife . . . oilcloth again. . . . Oh, I have got stuck at *oilcloth*. Is it a psychic vaudeville act? It sticks in my mind like a piece of glue . . . it is dirty. . . . [What shape?] Diamond shape . . . about one foot in diameter . . . it's like a rag. . . . I visualize it like a leaf dangling in the wind, it hangs on something under the sink . . . it's a dirty grey."

On the same day I had acquired a small box-shaped wooden footrest for use in my office and was quite pleased with the added comfort it meant to me. It had a polished surface and I asked my wife to procure a piece of linoleum or oilcloth cut to size with which to cover its top. I must confess that while listening to Fred's monotonous recital of obsessive thoughts my mind had wandered to the *oilcloth* which would have helped to relieve my feeling of fatigue at that time.

On relating the incident to my wife she supplied an additional piece of information. She had remembered an old sink-mat which she had replaced by a new one some time ago. Instead of throwing it away she had pushed it between a kitchen cabinet and the kitchen wall where it had remained since. She had been wondering whether, when cut to size, it would not serve the purpose of the piece of oilcloth I had asked for. I have to insert here that I knew nothing of the whereabouts of the sink-mat—although there is a possibility that lining the footrest with it might have crossed my mind independently of my wife. It will be noted that the patient's reference to a *dirty rag suspended* in some way from a sink and to its implied vertical position ("*dangling like a leaf* in the wind") suggests that here, again, my wife rather than I may have been the agent.

The last incident in the series occurred on July 7, 1949. The patient reported the following dream. "Some one was buying a wristwatch. She could not make up her mind whether to take the cheaper one or the more expensive one. She asked me to tell her which one to take. I told her the good qualities of both watches."

The buyer of the wristwatch reminded Fred of a German woman refugee, a psychiatrist's sister-in-law. She was promised a watch after the birth of her first child and she and her husband had consulted him about which watch to choose. He was pleased that they had turned to him and not to his father. This showed Fred that they had more confidence in his expert advice than in his father's. These associations led back to the transference relationship. The patient's dream obviously expressed his desire to be in the therapist's place, the therapist again representing his father.

This interpretation is further borne out by the psychological situation on my side of the picture. As it happened, on the evening preceding the dream I had a consultation with a new patient, a German refugee woman, whom I had first seen a week earlier. She was suffering from an acute exacerbation of an obsessive compulsive neurosis and could not make up her mind whether to start treatment with me. On July 7, 1949, she had come to see me again in great excitement. She had to choose between two apartments which were offered to her: a cheaper one on 97th Street and a more expensive one on 95th Street. I had to discuss with her in great detail the advantages and disadvantages of the two apartments and their respective locations. I got more involved in this discussion than I thought was advisable as a preliminary to analytic treatment and tried hard to avoid committing myself one way or the other.

It will be noted that Fred's dream seems to duplicate my own situation in five ways: (1) it contains a reference to an expert who is being consulted by a customer (patient); (2) the advice sought refers to two alternative choices, involving a cheaper and a more expensive item; (3) the pros and cons are equally divided between the two choices, making a detailed discussion of their qualities necessary; (4) in both cases it was a German lady who could not make up her mind; (5) both were "related" to a psychiatrist.

Nevertheless, it may well be objected that the four or five elements that are presumed to be common to both dream and corresponding real event are not specific enough to warrant a telepathic interpretation. It is at this point that the criterion of psychological significance or consistency can be resorted to in support of our thesis. The dreamer giving advice to his customer regarding jewellery quite obviously assumes the role of the therapist. He does exactly what the latter was called upon to do on the evening preceding the night on which the dream occurred. (My records show that the German lady had consulted me about her apartment as my last patient at 6 p.m.) Indeed, it has become sufficiently clear from the brief report of Fred's case that identification with the therapist had been an important feature of his attitude at that stage of the treatment.

Thus the telepathic interpretation of the dream is not only in good keeping with the orthodox analytical reading, it also furnishes additional clues in the same direction and, as it were, clinches the case. I may recall that in a number of dreams studied by J. Eisenbud,[33a,b,c] G. Pederson-Krag,[93a] and N. Fodor,[38] as well as in those discussed in the preceding chapters, it was only through proper appreciation of the telepathic factor involved that their latent meaning became apparent.

It may be well to sum up the five apparently telepathic incidents described in this section. In the first instance a telepathic factor seemed to be involved in the manifest content of the dream. Besides obvious references to the transference relationship, it contained three specific items that showed close correspondence to what had been my own emotionally coloured thoughts at the time the dream occurred. There was, first, reference to letting *light* and *air* into the *cellar*; second, to the *size* of the *window* through which that was to occur; thirdly, to my repressed desire of asking for a *favour* in connection with my wife's watch.

It will be noted that in this instance, as in the last dream of the series, it is the combination of several elements and their correspondence with a number of similarly interlacing elements in my own mind which is suggestive of its telepathic nature, even though the telepathic interpretation of the first dream is of lesser psychological significance to the over-all picture presented by the patient than in the last instance.

The three waking incidents are much more trivial and of lesser dynamic significance than the dreams reported here. To the sceptic Fred's unexpected reference to an air-conditioner, as yet not installed, may certainly appear less striking than to one who had already been expecting its arrival with impatience. (I hinted that the proposed installation of the unit had been a matter of a more intense preoccupation to me than I cared to admit in public.) The same is true for the incident involving my wife's new shoes. It will be recalled, however, that in this case not I but my wife had to be considered as the telepathic agent—provided that we are altogether satisfied with the telepathic nature of the case.

The fourth incident, trivial though it be, is unusual in that the patient himself was struck by his compulsive perseveration on so far-fetched an idea as an oilcloth dangling in the wind. He had the distinct feeling of its extraneous, heteropsychic origin, whereas he had remained unaware of the telepathic nature of earlier incidents. However, since by then (i.e. following the shoe incident) it was disclosed to him that a telepathic factor may have been intruding into our relationship, Fred's own puzzlement at what he called his psychic vaudeville act should be taken with a grain of salt. On the other hand, here again the coincidence with my own preoccupation with the same idea at the very same time is striking enough.

In trying to assess the pros and cons regarding the telepathic nature of the five observations described here, yet another factor has to be taken into consideration: their serial incidence within a limited space of time. I hinted that they occurred in the course of four or five sessions between the middle of May and the first week of July 1949, at a time when I had been seeing the patient twice a week. Two of the incidents occurred during the same session. Further, the serial incidence of apparently telepathic occurrences has to be considered against the fact that during the preceding twelve months of treatment no observation suggestive of telepathy had come to my notice in Fred's case.

Lastly, it should be recalled that the fifth telepathic incident, and its direct relevance to the psychodynamics revealed by Fred's analysis, lends added support to the telepathic interpretation of the whole series, even though the evidential value of the occurrences, taken by themselves, may be unequal and fall short of what I described as the criterion of uniqueness or specificity.

* * *

The present account would be incomplete without relating another observation which seems to have started off the series just discussed. On April 11, 1949, at the end of the session, the patient made a casual remark about warts on his right hand from which he had been suffering for several years. I was greatly interested at that time in the psychosomatic aspects of verrucae and had just been studying the pertinent literature. Actually, I had prepared a brief extract of references from the German literature for a friend who had started a research project concerned with suggestive and hypnotic treatment of warts. Fred's remark came too late for me to ask more particulars about them during that session. But the thought had crossed my mind that experiments of this kind would be well worth while in a patient with whom I had established good personal *rapport* and whose problems and personality structure had become so familiar to me. At the same time I dismissed the idea with a melancholy sigh, feeling as I did that it was to be one of the many research projects which for lack of time I had to leave for others to pursue. A week later, during the session on April 18, 1949, Fred reported a dream to the effect that "*the warts had come back.*"

When asked to elaborate on the scanty material contained in its manifest content, Fred said that he had two small warts on the volar aspect of the middle and ring fingers of his right hand and a big twin wart on the palm of his right hand. He claimed that the two warts on his fingers had disappeared during the past week and that only the twin wart on his right palm had remained. Fred showed the places on which, according to his account, the warts had been located prior to their disappearance. I could see what appeared to be superficial epithelial defects on the spots indicated by the patient. They may or may not have been the last traces of what was left of the warts.

Since, unfortunately, I had missed the opportunity of convincing myself of the existence of the warts in time, I sought to obtain an affidavit from Fred's mother concerning his statement. The affidavit, as reproduced below,* is unsatisfac-

* This note is to verify the fact that my son Fred had three warts, one on the palm of his right hand and two adjacent to each other on his second and first fingers of his right hand which disappeared during his analytical treatment sometime in April, May, or June 1949. I can remember these warts for at least three years previous to 1949.—Mrs. L.

tory inasmuch as it is indefinite as to the exact time of the disappearance and conflicting as to the location of the warts. The whole wart incident cannot, therefore, be regarded as anything like scientific proof regarding an assumed telepathic effect of my emotionally coloured—yet repressed—therapeutic motivations aiming at their suggestive treatment. The possibility cannot be ruled out that the warts were no longer there when the patient first mentioned them to me. Further, it is possible that, despite my failure to verbalize in any way my interest in the matter I may unwittingly have imparted some inkling of it to the patient and that Fred, in turn, may have unconsciously connected certain expectations with his remark which set into motion the chain of psychosomatic events that ultimately led to the disappearance of the warts—without a telepathic factor being involved in the process.

However that may be, it goes without saying that the described incident itself may well have provided just that emotional impetus in the mind of both therapist and patient which, from all we know about the general predisposing factors of telepathy, may have paved the way for the subsequent series of more conclusive telepathic incidents.

* * *

What, then, is the significance of these observations? If we are satisfied with their telepathic nature they seem to confirm the formulations put forward in the preceding chapters regarding predisposing factors which are conducive to telepathy in the psychoanalytic situation. In Fred's case the stage was set by my own emotionally coloured preoccupation with what—rightly or wrongly—I first took for a telepathic reaction involving the disappearance of warts. Even though it may have been a largely mistaken notion on my part, it appears to have touched off the subsequent series of real incidents.

A further factor may have been the patient's anxiety to co-operate with the therapist, to please him with the production of just such analytic material as he "intuitively" felt would arouse his special interest. Fred had been told that the treatment might draw to a close sooner than expected. From his earlier reading on psychoanalysis he had learned that the patient was supposed to remember and to bring up as many early childhood recollections as possible. He had actually made repeated references to that effect during that period of treatment. Fred also knew of the therapist's interest in the problem of telepathy and had actually read his book on the subject before coming for treatment. Although no mention of the matter had been made during the further course of analysis, it may well be that the wart incident—which I had discussed with the patient in terms of a possible case of "autosuggestion"—had evoked in him the desire to do better next time at what Fred himself had called his psychic vaudeville act.

As far as the recall of early infantile material is concerned, the patient had produced no new recollections and continued his acting out on an oral and anal sadistic level for several more weeks. In short, Fred passed into a new period of resistance, indicating that he was not ready as yet to terminate treatment. Viewed against the background of analytic resistance it may well be that offering telepathic (i.e. heteropsychic) experiences of an inoffensive nature had served him as a convenient substitute for other material which he could not face.

Closer study of the patient's productions at that time shows, however, that the isolated telepathic incidents described were in effect interspersed with material of just that more offensive order. I indicated that some of the incidents occurred while Fred was reciting his compulsive thoughts referring to kicking, biting, sucking, defaecating, etc., even though this was not accompanied by the corresponding affects. It will be noted that this dissociation of affect, well known in compulsion neurotics, is at the same time a characteristic feature of the schizophrenic patient. This is all the more significant if we recall at this point my earlier observations about occasional telepathic occurrences in the associational context of deteriorated schizophrenics. The telepathic reactions seen in this group are in many respects similar to those produced by the compulsion neurotic discussed here. An example taken from my book *Telepathy and Medical Psychology* may illustrate the point. The rambling "word salad" of one of the patients, a girl of twenty-one, contained striking allusions to my thoughts connected with her *Jewish appearance*; with the idea of *make-up* which had struck me in a patient confined to the refractory ward; to a *bottle of ether* with which I had been experimenting at that time, etc. All this was thrown into a chaotic welter of deeply regressional material of autopsychic origin that formed the overwhelming majority of her utterances.

What, then, is the common denominator in the compulsion neurotic discussed here and the schizophrenic described in my earlier observations? Obviously, it is in both instances the removal of a barrier which permits the emergence of heteropsychic experiences. In Fred's case their breakthrough is due to the temporary weakening of the barrier, affecting only limited areas of the ego. It was presumably helped by the release of early infantile material encouraged at that period of the treatment.

Expressing the relation of autopsychic to heteropsychic material as in the fraction below, it could be stated that in Fred's case its ratio is considerably > 1.

$$\frac{\text{autopsychic}}{\text{heteropsychic}} = > 1$$

In the advanced schizophrenic, by contrast, the breakdown of the barrier affects all areas of the patient's ego; it is of a global nature. What happens in these cases is not merely a limited intrusion of primitive regressional material; the patient's ego is totally engulfed by the "Return of the Repressed." But it is interesting to note that here, again, the demonstrably heteropsychic elements are usually but a fraction of the total repressed material that breaks through the boundaries of the ego. I may add by way of a footnote only that in the genuine "psychic" the hypothetical ratio

$$\frac{\text{autopsychic}}{\text{heteropsychic}}$$

experiences may be considerably smaller. If we can give credence to reports about certain spectacular trance manifestations in a few highly gifted mediums, it may occasionally become < 1.

There is another important aspect of the psychodynamics of

telepathy which is brought out by our patient. I indicated that in two of the telepathic incidents described Fred's telepathic sensitiveness was not confined to influences emanating from myself. He seemed to reflect emotionally coloured elements which were either exclusively or preponderantly derived from my wife. If this is true we have to realize that the psychoanalytic situation, despite its closely guarded privacy, does not operate in a watertight compartment, as it were. The patient-doctor relationship, besides being determined by the dynamics of transference and countertransference—including the occasional two-way leakage of heteropsychic material—may be further complicated by telepathic leakage from other persons: in the present case by leakage from one who was, of course, known to the patient to be in close relationship with the present writer.

I may recall here my discussion of the identical problem in relation to telepathic influences that may be brought to bear upon a schizophrenic patient from outside the controlled hospital environment.[32] But it goes without saying that in the absence of sufficient information as to the personalities of such potential external agents that may force their way into the psychoanalytic situation, there is no easy way by which further systematic research in this direction could proceed at the present moment. The telepathic leakage seen in Fred's case shows, however, that the therapist must always be aware of such a possibility. Indeed, he should do well to realize that the classical concept of the doctor-patient relationship operating within an isolated system according to the formula transference-countertransference is no longer tenable. It has to be replaced by the concept of a vastly expanded field of heteropsychic influences which may, or may not, impinge on both patient and therapist and thus modify the psychoanalytic situation—if not our outlook on the world at large. This, however, is a problem the discussion of which has been reserved for a later chapter.

CHAPTER VI

Fred Has Another Telepathic Dream

THE incidents discussed in the preceding chapter were not the last numbers in what Fred described as his psychic vaudeville act. It will be recalled that the incidents occurred in the course of a few sessions towards the end of about one year's analysis. This phase was followed by a marked improvement in the patient's condition and it was decided that his treatment should be interrupted for a prolonged trial period.

Fred's improvement was maintained for about one year, during which time he had remained in touch with the therapist. It was followed by recurrence of some of his obsessive thoughts so that resumption of treatment was agreed upon. The beginning of this second treatment period was ushered in by a new wave of anal-sadistic fantasies produced in the patient's free associations. Aggressive tendencies towards both the therapist and his wife dominated the picture, alternating with a veiled homosexual trend. On the other hand he showed a marked passive, submissive attitude, expressing his unconscious identification with his mother. At the same time he put the therapist in his father's place and involved him in homosexual fantasies. Or else, he would indulge in veiled incestuous daydreams connected with his mother.

In the second month of the renewed period of treatment Fred reported the following dream:

"My mother's room was dark and something was wrong with the light. The room was the vestibule in her apartment, adjoining the porch. I was fixing wires or pieces of string attached to each other. I pulled the strings so that the light would work again. I had the impression that the room was changed or that something had to be remodelled in it. I had to crawl into the place, I don't know why. It had a floor sloping towards the centre. In the middle there was a drain-pipe, perhaps to collect rainwater. I found it strange to see a drain-pipe in the middle of a room."

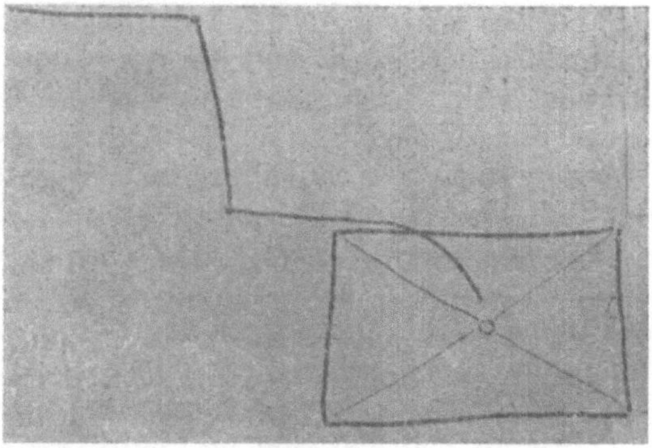

FIG. 4.—Mother's room with drain-pipe. Tracing of Fred's pencil sketch.

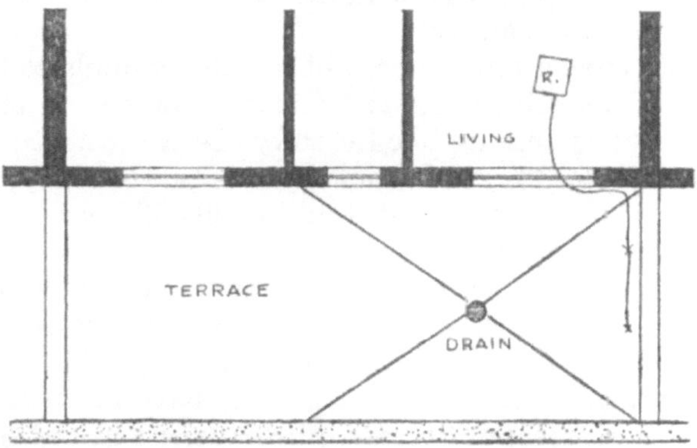

FIG. 5.—Floor plan showing living room, radio with aerial cord, sloping terrace floor and drain-pipe.

The patient's sketch reproduced above shows the rectangular vestibule with the drain-pipe in the centre and to the left the outlines of what he described as his mother's porch, with the staircase leading up to it. It will be noted that the chief emphasis of the drawing is placed on the rectangular box-shaped vestibule. The zig-zag line on the right is drawn with equal emphasis. It represents the electric wire or cord which the patient was supposed to fix for his mother. The drawing also indicates two points on which the cord is fixed to something—the patient could not tell to what.

As usual Fred's associations to this dream were influenced by his previous analysis. He connected the dark room into which he had to crawl with his mother's womb. Accordingly, the drain pipe and the cord stood for the birth canal, umbilical cord, etc. This in turn was closely connected with anal and urethral fantasies, due to early infantile confusion regarding the various body openings. The wires also reminded him of an electric shock he had received at the age of eight when he and his sister had played with the wire connection of a Christmas tree. Earlier he had once put his finger into an electric socket and also had received an electric shock. Sex play with his sister and her friends and fear that he might be caught by his father were his next associations. Another trend of thought led from the drain-pipe to memories of being bathed with his sister in the same bath tub.

After digression into a chain of largely compulsive fantasies, Fred added an afterthought: "Today I wanted to tell you a phony story; something like the story about the air-conditioner I told you a year ago, so I would please you. Actually, after the last session I thought what it would be like if I were to concoct a new telepathic story for you."

While giving his account the patient had noted my keen interest in his report. He saw I was writing down word for word what he said. At times I would interrupt him, asking him to repeat a sentence or two. This may have been one of the reasons for his facetious remarks interspersed in the rest of his compulsive utterances. The fact is that his facetious reference to the possible telepathic implication of his dream was not mistaken. As it happened, the evening before the dream occurred, on September 14, 1950, a radio repairman had been in my apartment to repair a chairside model radio set which had recently broken down. The man said there was not much wrong with it. All that was needed was a new outdoor aerial so as to improve reception of FM. He had also tightened some screws to secure the power supply. All this I learned from my wife on coming home from the office the same night. She had already purchased the aerial cord and asked me to attach it to the set according to the repairman's advice. As seen in Fig. 5, the radio is situated in the living room which opens through a french door and two windows to the terrace belonging to our apartment. I led the wires through the open door on to the terrace, turning them in a right angle to the left and fastening them by drawing-pins to a wooden box in the corner. From there I turned the wires in another right angle to the left and

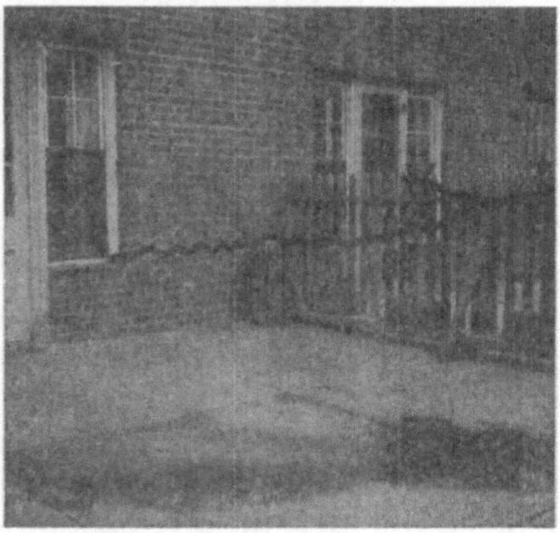

FIG. 6.—The therapist's terrace with drain-pipe and radio aerial.

fastened them at two places to a small wooden fence separating our part of the terrace from our next-door neighbour. (This layout can also be compared with Fig. 2, p. 42, showing the floor plan of the apartment in its relation to the terrace two years earlier, that is, at a time when the wooden fence had not yet been erected. It will be recalled that this situation figured in Ruth's dream discussed in Chapter III.)

As can be seen in Fig. 6 the terrace itself has a concrete floor sloping toward the middle. Slightly off centre there is a drain-pipe to collect rainwater. I must add here that the wires constituting the aerial were not in one piece; they were fastened together like pieces of string at points indicated by the crosses in the floor plan. I had also to do much pulling of the wires during the whole procedure, partly because they were not gripped tight enough by the two antenna screws, partly because they had to be conducted outside the door under the door-mat. As can be readily seen from this description I am no expert in fixing broken-down radios. On the contrary, the job was done with considerable fumbling and fussing and was only persisted in because both the present writer and his family were most anxious to have the radio in working order so as to be able to enjoy a particular concert which was to be on the FM programme that evening.

There was another difficulty, though not of a technical kind, connected with installing the aerial. My landlord had made provisions for a big master antenna on the roof of our apartment house for the use of which he charged a considerable sum of money. The installation of any other outdoor aerials by tenants was prohibited. I was rather reluctant to break this rule, however unfair I found it to be. Since my wife, however, had already taken the first step in defying the "law," I felt I had to go on with the job though with pangs of conscience—or to be more specific, with some anxiety about the way the superintendent would react to my breaking the landlord's rules.

On comparing the manifest content of the patient's dream with the situation on my side of the picture on the night the dream occurred, a number of corresponding features can again be detected. There is, first, the *motif* of "changing or remodelling something" that was wrong in the room. Secondly, there is reference to electric wires which had to be fixed. Thirdly, there is a specific remark about strings that had to be attached to each other. Fourthly, there is the description of a sloping floor with, fifth, a drain-pipe in its centre. Sixth and seventh, there are more details as to the way in which the wires were conducted through the door, twice bent in a right angle and fastened to "something" at two places.

This combination of seven or eight distinctive features in both dream and reality, in conjunction with the temporal coincidence, is striking enough to be suggestive of telepathy. Indeed, some of the details contained in the manifest content of the dream illustrate what I described as the telepathic tracer effect better than any of the incidents reviewed in earlier chapters. In short, the dream described here seems to meet the criterion of specificity or uniqueness as well as can be expected from any spontaneous incident of this type.

On the face of it the criterion of psychological significance which, I stated, may serve as an important added argument in favour of the telepathic interpretation, is less obvious. It will be recalled that the symbolic interpretation of Fred's dream in terms of his wish to return to the security of his mother's womb and of a gratification of repressed anal tendencies had become clear to the dreamer himself. Again, the wires reminded him of sex play and incestuous wishes connected with his sister—and of the punishment which may ensue. All this seems adequate to account for the greater part of the manifest content of the dream. Unless we make due allowance for its telepathic aspect, however, we are at a loss to understand some of the specific details featured in the dream; that is, the bizarre condensation of his mother's room with an open place having a *sloping floor* and a *drain-pipe* in the centre is only explicable if we assume that the patient succeeded in catching a telepathic glimpse of some of my own preoccupations on the same night. In effect, as soon as we make allowance for the telepathic implications of the dream we are faced with a new aspect of its latent meaning.

What, then, are the implications of its telepathic interpretations? First and foremost, the patient seems to be watching the activities of the therapist and his wife on the night the dream occurred. At the same time he seems anxious to convey to him by his dream that he knows "all" about him and his wife. This has to be viewed against the fact that references to the primal scene have loomed large in his compulsive productions at this period of the treatment. In other words, the dream seems to express the patient's wish to become part of and to participate in the therapist's life according to the neurotic equation

therapist	=	the patient's father
the therapist's wife	=	the patient's mother or sister.

The dream obviously fulfils that part of Fred's repressed desires. But how does he escape the anxiety that is usually attached to the gratification of such wishes?

We have to assume that in this respect he is aided by the familiar device of distortion, symbolic representation and condensation, characteristic of both the dream and the telepathic process. A further clue to that effect can be found when we cast a brief glance at the psychodynamics as they existed on my side of the picture.

I hinted that in view of existing regulations I was reluctant to install the outdoor aerial purchased by my wife. This reluctance can be traced back to three very good reasons. First, it was due to the hesitation of the ordinary law-abiding citizen to break the "law." Secondly, it was connected with the painful memory of an argument a few years earlier with the same landlord who issued the anti-aerial regulation. In that argument I felt I had gone too far in expressing a sense of "righteous" indignation over an otherwise trivial matter that had come up between us. To make matters worse, it was now I who laid myself open to the reproach of violating the honour code. A third reason leads to more significant aspects. On a deeper level the incident may be connected with guilt feelings of my own over breaking certain taboos and in engaging in "forbidden" activities with my wife, duplicating, as it were, the dreamer's incestuous fantasies.

Had the patient caught a telepathic glimpse of my own repressed intrapsychic conflicts? Did he derive some solace from the fact that he was not the only one who had "broken the law" and that he had actually caught me redhanded violating the rules issued by a figure in authority? If so, this may well have served to allay Fred's anxiety over his forbidden fantasies involving my wife as a mother substitute, as well as diminishing his fear of retribution for watching what, to him, had amounted to a representation of the primal scene—if not to the repetition of the Original Sin itself.

These reflections should go far to show that here, again, allowance made for the telepathic aspects of the dream serves as a decisive aid towards a proper understanding of its deeper meaning. In this way, and in this way only, are we able to fit it in with the patient's neurotic problem in general and with his attitude in the transference relationship in particular. If this is true the telepathic appreciation of the dream is in good keeping with what I described as the criterion of psychological significance or consistency with an expanded and revised system of dynamic psychiatry as it is aimed at in the present study.

These considerations, however, do not exhaust the psychodynamic implications of Fred's dream. The patient's facetious remarks on noticing my unusual interest in his account should call attention to another aspect of the telepathic process. Viewed from the conventional psychoanalytic point of view it could be stated that Fred's little "dig" at me was due to irritation over seeing me involved in an issue which had little to do with his personal problem. Sensitive as he was on that score, he had felt left out and neglected. But it will be recalled that, on his own admission, he had already toyed with the idea of taunting me at the end of the preceding session. This would indicate that Fred's attitude was nothing but another manifestation of his resistance to the therapist or, more precisely, of what psychoanalysis calls the patient's transference resistance. In any case, Fred was anxious to make me understand that whatever striking material he may have produced in his analytic session was not really intended to support my pet scientific hypothesis—or if it did so, this was merely due to his generously concocting or dreaming up stories to please "father." If he had sensed that he had in actual fact obliged the therapist by supplying material of that very kind, he sought to redress himself now by denying its validity.

On a still deeper level, his transference resistance may have served another purpose. It may well be that Fred, feeling threatened by what he himself had sensed as an intrusion of heteropsychic material into his ego, was anxious to reinforce his defences against his telepathic sensitiveness, much in the same way as we know that patients may seek to protect themselves against the threat of positive transference on the therapist by reinforcing their ordinary ego defences. As it happened, however, Fred's resistance had not been strong enough to prevent the telepathic incidents described—obviously because his voyeuristic desire, combined with his need to reach out for my extra attention and approval, was stronger than the ego defences militating against the occurrence of telepathy.

Another feature of the dream reviewed here emerges on comparing its manifest content with some of the dreams discussed in previous chapters. There is, first, Ruth's case described in Chapter III. It will be recalled that the manifest content of her dream contained references to my apartment, its layout and furnishings. Yet the striking fact is that Fred seemed to be doing much better in capturing various details (e.g. particulars referring to the terrace floor) than Ruth had been able to do. Put in this way, our formulation admittedly implies the unorthodox assumption that Fred had actually been trying to compete with Ruth's telepathic exploits and sought to outstrip her in producing a dream of greater evidential value. In studying Fred's whole attitude there can be little doubt that an exhibitionistic need to get "good marks" in his analysis has indeed been a characteristic feature of his mental make-up. During the first treatment period he had repeatedly referred to his "psychic vaudeville act." He was in open competition with his friend Ronald H. whose telepathic dream was discussed in Chapter IV. In turn, Ronald, who had entered analysis about one year after him, exhibited much the same competitive attitude toward his senior colleague. All this may well have served as an added incentive for our dreamer to loosen the barriers against the potential intrusion of telepathic material into his dream life, even though we have seen that at the same time he did not altogether relinquish his guards against telepathic sensitiveness in general.

CHAPTER VII

When the Therapist Has a Dream

so far we have discussed one type of telepathic dream only: dreams in which the therapist was the agent and the patient the percipient. From all we know about the nature of the telepathic process and of therapeutic *rapport* in general, it can safely be expected, however, that the therapist may be equally affected by telepathic influences emanating from the patient—provided that his own resistance is not too strongly set against them and provided that he is at all prepared to pay attention to the *psi* factor entering the treatment situation on his side of the picture.

The dream which will presently be discussed was precipitated by an incident in which Fred L. and Ronald H., the two friends and rivals whose dreams were discussed in the preceding chapters, were involved. First, the dream: I found myself travelling with my patient Ronald H. on the platform of a tram-car. It was of a distinctly European type such as I have been used to seeing in Prague and Vienna before the war. Ronald passed a German newspaper to me to read. I knew it was a Berlin or possibly German-language Prague newspaper. Then the scene shifted and I was put in a humiliating situation of which it is enough to say in the present connection that it was of an undisguised anal nature.

The dream was so vivid and its emotional impact upon me so intense that I did an unusual thing on awakening. I wrote it down verbatim in Ronald's case sheet strongly suspecting its telepathic nature. I may add that I cannot remember ever having dreamt of Ronald before and that references to any one of my patients are of the greatest rarity in my dream life. Ronald opened his session on the same morning with an unusually sharp attack against me. The night before (that is, on the night of my dream) he had been visiting in Fred's house and learned from him that I had written a medical certificate for Fred which was of great help to him in relation to business difficulties. Ronald disapproved of his friend for having asked for such a certificate and got into a heated argument with him about it. Ronald, still indignant, wanted to carry on the debate in our session. He reproached me for having done Fred an utterly undeserved favour. Fred, he stated, was unfair in asking for the certificate and my giving in to him amounted to aiding and abetting unfair practices of which he had long before suspected his rival. Fred, as a Jew, should have been particularly anxious to avoid such practices and the same responsibility should have been incumbent on me: "This is just what you hear the Nazis are whispering about when the chips are down and you, of all people, have helped him in pulling such tricks."

Ronald's attack on me was in striking contrast to his customary polite and submissive behaviour. While in the past he had exhibited marked positive transference, identifying the therapist with his greatly admired and beloved father, and repressing all the hostility against the latter, he now suddenly reversed his position in passionate denunciation and open invective. There could be no doubt that he deeply resented the apparent favouritism shown by the father figure to Fred whom he in turn regarded as the personification of his older brother with whom he had unsuccessfully vied for his father's favours in his childhood years.

From the psychoanalytic point of view Ronald's behaviour toward me was thus a typical instance of acting out his childhood conflict in relation to the Oedipal situation and sibling rivalry. This is also borne out by the fact that as a result of my interpretation the situation was soon under control and the therapeutic relationship between patient and analyst restored.

What, then, is the connection between my dream and the incident just described? On weighing the potential telepathic implications of the dream itself we have first to make due allowance for its intense emotional impact upon the dreamer himself. Never before have I been so impressed by a dream of my own as to make an entry of it in the patient's case history to whom it referred. To this has to be added the correspondence between the identity of the person featured in the dream and an actual event occurring on the night of the dream in which an irate Ronald had been the major protagonist. This may well be taken as an example of a telepathic incident meeting with the criterion of specificity if not uniqueness.

The rest of the manifest content appearing in the dream requires more comment. I already mentioned my own associations in connection with the tram-car. It reminded me of post-war Europe which I had visited in 1945. Again, the Berlin or Prague newspaper recalled the violent anti-semitic campaign which had swept over all the German Press during the Second World War and whose late reverberations I could still feel during my post-war stay in Prague. However, no possible connection between anti-semitic newspaper comment and Ronald's attitude had occurred to me prior to his outburst in the session on the following day. He was Roman Catholic of Polish descent, but held liberal views and was at times in open rebellion against his own background and religious denomination.

The humiliating situation in which I had found myself in the second part of the dream brought my earlier self-searching in connection with the dream described in the preceding chapter into mind. It will be recalled that I was wondering about the relevance of Fred's dream to guilt feelings attached to remnants of certain pregenital conflicts of my own. Other, less specific, features of my countertransference upon both patients are of lesser significance and need not be discussed in the present connection. The important point is that learning of Ronald's outburst against me on the night of my dream helps to fill the gap in our understanding of both its manifest content and latent meaning.

Obviously, Ronald's passing the Berlin or Prague newspaper to me indicates the violent anti-semitic colouring of his negative transference while the humiliating anal situation in which I found myself in the dream has to be interpreted as my own reaction to his attack, accusing me of favouritism towards his rival so as to gain financial (i.e. anal) benefits for myself. Other aspects of the dream are too personal to lend themselves for public discussion.

It will be noted that no words were spoken throughout the whole dream as though I had sought to silence my accuser at least on the verbal level in order to allay my anxiety aroused by his reproaches and conveyed to me in a telepathic way. In this respect the dream thus served its well-known purpose of protecting the sleeper's ego from the disturbing effect of inner tension, conflict, or discomfort as postulated by Freud.

In other respects, however, the dream shows several features which distinguish it from the dreams discussed so far. First and foremost, in this instance it is the therapist and not the patient whose emotional response to the transference situation is reflected telepathically by the dream. There was no conscious intention on the part of the therapist to "oblige" anybody—not even himself—by producing such a dream. If there had been such an intention, it had in any case been utterly unsuccessful in the past. Despite all my interest in the problem of telepathy there are barely more than two or three telepathic dreams of my own in my records. My dream life on the whole has certainly been subject to the principle of frustrated volition.

What, then, accounts for my unusual telepathic susceptibility in the present instance? Obviously it is the sheer violence of the patient's emotional reaction to a symbolic betrayal by the beloved father figure which must, at least in part, be held responsible for the incident described. It was this betrayal which had aroused Ronald's iconoclastic wrath so that he was ready to tear down his idol and to strike at its most vulnerable spots. This attitude may have met halfway, as it were, my own unconscious guilt feelings over whatever favours I had bestowed on Fred in preference to his friend—to say nothing of guilt feelings pertaining to deeper levels.

Be that as it may, the importance of the dream described here goes far beyond its implications as far as psychodynamics of the telepathic process are concerned. It shows that regardless of his conscious goals and motivations the therapist's own ego may be laid open to the impact of heteropsychic material emanating from his patient. This is rarely brought out with such dramatic force as in the dream discussed in this chapter.

Here again, however, it is from a few striking observations that we can draw conclusions as to many subtler ways in which *psi* may be involved in the therapeutic situation and in interpersonal relationships in general.

But it should be noted at this point that occasional telepathic dreams dreamt by the therapist are not the only clues pointing to his direct "intuitive" sensitivity to the patient's mental content, conscious or unconscious. Elsewhere[32] I mentioned an observation of my own in which such a communication was suggested by a waking incident showing an unmistakable tracer effect. One of my patients, a man of twenty-four, repeatedly mentioned *Miss B.* whose faithlessness, he said, was the chief cause of his depression. He never gave me her full name. One day he recounted a dream which again centred on the person of the faithless *Miss B.* His account was highly emotional. I tried to summarize the dream: "There is one block of facts . . ." I started to say when the patient butted in with visible indignation. "Please don't mention this word . . . her name is *Miss Block*, I hate to hear it."

I had never before used the phrase "block of facts" in a similar context. Indeed, its use at that moment was quite out of place and might well be attributed to a slip of my tongue—but to one occasioned by repressed content originating from the patient. Similar incidents, when occurring in the absence of tracer elements, are usually described as the analyst's intuitive reaction to the patient's unconscious. The following is the typical observation of this kind.

Mr. Z., a man of forty-three, has been my patient for a year and a half. He was suffering from a compulsion neurosis and various hypochondriacal fears. Considerable progress had been made in his treatment and I felt we had reached the stage when the resolution of the transference relationship should become our prime objective. One morning I decided to drop a hint as to the need for winding up and ultimately terminating the treatment. The patient, somewhat taken aback, voiced his objections. The rest of the hour was taken up by discussing his manoeuvres to find substitute analysts to lean on in case he should have to give me up. He played cards with his neighbour, a general practitioner; his steady golfing companion was a doctor friend, and he was a frequent guest in the house of an uncle, a laryngologist. At the end of the session, on second thought, as it were, Mr. Z. reported the following dream: "I am afraid my manufacturer will stop supplying the merchandise I need. I hope he won't. I could get really rich if the supply continued. I could have a gorgeous house, a sailing yacht, girls and all that. But I also thought he might cut the production. Therefore I made a chemical analysis of his product so I will be able to manufacture it myself. I'll call it the improved so-and-so product."

The meaning of the dream is obvious. The dreamer reassures himself as to his ability to stand on his own feet and to continue with his own "analysis" in case his therapist should terminate the treatment and "cut off the supply" of emotional security derived from it. But how are we to account for the fact that Mr. Z. related the dream at the end of a session which I myself had ushered in with the very suggestion which provided the principal theme of the dream? Had both the therapist and the patient arrived independently at the identical conclusion (i.e. that the treatment should be terminated) simply because both had taken their cues from the same set of premises? If so, the coincidence of the therapist's remarks with the latent meaning expressed by the dream has to be regarded as the result of unconscious rational inferences showing admittedly striking identity as to timing and content. Such an interpretation, in any case, would dispense with the need of resorting to the *psi* factor to account for an unusual feat of intuition.

In the present context, however, telepathy operating between therapist and patient seems to be at least an equally justifiable explanatory hypothesis. It can rightly be argued that a telepathic factor has been involved in the very process by which the assumed unconscious inferences had led to identical conclusions at the same time—leaving open the question as to who has been playing the part of the agent and who the part of the percipient. It is true that the absence of unmistakable tracer elements considerably weakens the merits of a telepathic interpretation. But this is in effect the case in most instances usually described in terms of intuition—whatever the term is meant to indicate.

There is another, not less intriguing, problem which is posed by the dream discussed here. Accepting for argument's sake its telepathic interpretation, it can well be asked whether it was the therapist's "intuition" which anticipated the latent meaning of a dream the patient was just about to relate or whether it was the patient who had caught a telepathic glimpse ahead of time of the therapist's intention to deal with the same problem? In short, it might be asked whether the telepathic incident described was due to telepathy pure and simple, or to what is known as precognitive telepathy operating either from the therapist to the patient or from the patient to the therapist. Needless to say, in the case discussed here the question cannot be decided one way or the other. But it serves as a convenient point of departure for the discussion of the problem of time in general in relation to telepathy, precognitive, post-cognitive or otherwise, which for reasons that should presently become apparent is bound to come up in our argument.

CHAPTER VIII

*Precognition in Dreams?**

IT is a generally accepted principle of the scientific method that the lesser the degree of credibility of a hypothesis, the greater must be the weight of evidence on which the hypothesis is based. Applying this principle to the telepathy hypothesis we should be expected to supply a vast and indeed overwhelming number of detailed observations in its favour.

Yet the history of science shows that it is not the number of isolated data, however striking they may be, but their assemblage within a system of mutually consistent generalizations and explanatory hypotheses which carries conviction.

Have we reached the point at which the reader is satisfied with the factual evidence presented here so that more can be gained by a tentative evaluation of the material than by the further amassing of isolated data? One might be inclined to answer this question in the affirmative—provided that the type of observations discussed so far was the only one which came within our purview. Such observations as the presumptively telepathic incident which was briefly discussed in the previous chapter show, however, that unfortunately this is not the case.

Telepathy has been defined as awareness by one person of another person's mental processes without the aid of sensory channels. It will be noted that this formulation makes no reference to the problem of temporal coincidence of the two sets of mental events concerned. Yet the fact is that the notion of temporal coincidence, whatever this may be taken to indicate, is tacitly implied by the customary definition. But when and under what circumstances are we justified in describing two sets of events, mental or physical, as contemporaneous? The early workers in psychical research were satisfied on this score when the events in question occurred "at the same time"

* Published in part in *Psychoan. Review*, 38, 1951.

as measured by the position of the hands of two synchronized clocks, i.e. when the time lag between them was not more than a specified number of minutes or hours.

However, even before the advent of relativistic physics, shaking as it does the foundations of the Newtonian concept of absolute time, this has been a procedure beset by many difficulties. How, in the absence of proper experimental safeguards, should the exact timing of two geographically remote physical events be carried out and what is it that constitutes such well-defined physical events? "Simultaneity" is still more difficult to define where two series of presumptively corresponding mental events are concerned which cannot, for obvious reasons, be strictly pinpointed on the imaginary time continuum. The problem can best be illustrated by a fictitious example of prescience or precognitive telepathy taken from Shakespeare's *Macbeth*.

The three witches on the heath, we are told, prophesied to Macbeth that he would be "Thane of Glamis, Thane of Cawdor and King hereafter." Macbeth resolutely rejects this idea:

> Whose horrid image does unfix my hair
> and makes my seated heart knock at my ribs.

But from then onward the seed put into his mind by the witches' prophecy grows into the tragic deeds that lead to his doom and ultimate undoing with the inevitability of the ancient Greek tragedy.

Now it may well be stated that this alleged prophecy was largely due to telepathic sensitiveness on the part of the weird sisters to Macbeth's unconscious desire to take the place of his rival and to slay, if need be, Duncan, the fatherly king. Yet if we accept this interpretation another question arises. One might rightly ask: How long, then, has the seed of Macbeth's savage ambition been lying dormant in his unconscious? Can it legitimately be described as a mental event present in his mind then and there when he found himself face to face with the three witches on the "blasted heath"? Or is it more appropriate to assume that he was not only unaware at that time of his unconscious desires but that he did not, as a matter of fact, even "dream" of the horrible things that lay in store for him in the future? In short, it may be questioned whether the witches' utterances were of a precognitive nature or due to telepathy "pure and simple."

Obviously, this question is difficult to decide in a hypothetical case that springs from the creative artist's imagination only; but we have seen in the previous chapter that much the same difficulty arises whenever we are confronted with a concrete clinical observation. The early workers in psychical research did not get far beyond stating the existence of the problem. They found that in the majority of their observations the actual incident either preceded or followed its telepathic perception rather than being strictly contemporaneous with it. Since measurable simultaneity was in any case difficult to establish they sought to circumvent this stumbling block by postulating an arbitrary time span of twenty-four hours within which two corresponding sets of mental events were to be considered in terms of simultaneous telepathy. Cases in which a specifiable period of time seemed to have lapsed between the incident and its presumably telepathic perception could then easily be attributed to a latency period during which the telepathic message remained subliminal or dormant, as it were, in the unconscious. But there were recurrent reports in the literature of psychical research describing observations in which the apparently telepathic incident had preceded the actual mental event. Some of the observations described in *Phantasms of the Living*[52] are of this type, and the reader familiar with the pertinent literature will recall Dunne's *An Experiment with Time*[31] which contains accounts of a great number of apparently precognitive dreams.

Observations like these cannot be disregarded in the present connection, however embarrassing they may be to an investigator brought up in the traditions of our current scientific scheme of thinking to which alleged foreknowledge of future events is still more difficult to accept than telepathy of the ordinary kind.

* * *

A case in point is the following instance of an apparently precognitive dream. It was reported by a male patient, Mr. T., aged thirty-eight, suffering from anxiety hysteria. Working as a floor manager in a big department store he was greatly inconvenienced by severe anxiety attacks whenever he travelled in a bus or the underground. More recently the attacks came over him also on crossing busy streets, in cinemas, in restaurants, and even at the fountain counter of his store. Analysis showed that Mr. T.'s symptoms served as a defensive mechanism directed against unconscious homosexual impulses which were aggravated in the phobic situations.

After initial difficulties the treatment made good progress. The patient had gradually become able to face repressed material without untoward reactions but had still remained restricted in his movements and in need of a "bodyguard" when travelling. His dreams showed unmistakable evidence of positive transference. At that time—in the fourth month of psychotherapy, consisting of three sessions a week—he produced the following dream which is quoted verbatim from my records.

"I was in the store. There was a guy who apparently worked for us. I had the feeling he was after something, ready to hold up the place. He had a large flip-open knife, opening it, closing it, suggesting he was a dangerous fellow. I got scared, called for Mr. X. and Mr. Y. to catch the man. I myself retreated into the telephone booth to call the police to get him. All of a sudden the whole situation seemed to have dissolved. The guy was sitting there; I was talking to him. It was a more friendly conversation. He took out the knife, flipped it open. It was not large any more—just half an inch or maybe an inch long. I thought how foolish it was to be afraid of the knife. It was not nearly as dangerous as it looked, it was very small."

The patient's associations made the homosexual nature of the hold-up situation obvious. The phallic symbolism of the knife needs no further elaboration. The two men mentioned in the dream were his colleagues who used to accompany him in the underground or bus. His call for the police stood for his invoking the help of the therapist in warding off his unconscious homosexual impulses. Again, the sudden change of the scene in which the large knife turned out to be quite small and harmless was an obvious reference to the therapeutic progress made, to his feeling that he was no longer afraid of his repressed homosexual tendencies. It was at this point that I felt the time had come to offer him an interpretation and to advise him to try actively to overcome his phobia. Mr. T. left greatly relieved and I had the impression that an important step had been made towards his recovery.

The next session was two days later, on the morning of November 7, 1947. The patient was some five minutes late. He reported with an embarrassed smile that on getting on the bus he saw a "coloured fellow" sitting next to him at the back of the bus take a knife out of his pocket and open it quite unconcerned. It was a little pen-knife, just like the one in the second half of the dream. The patient added, "I felt quite uneasy, ready to get panicky any time, keeping an eye on him. Then he took an apple out of his pocket, cut it, and started calmly eating it."

Mr. T. gave this account greatly amazed at the apparent correspondence of parts of his dream and the subsequent event on the bus. "The knife," he added, "was like taken out of the dream. But, please, don't think that I am suffering from hallucinations. Never has a similar thing happened to me before." He further added that he had missed the previous bus by a few seconds. That was the reason for being late at the session.

Remarkable though the existing points of resemblance between the two sets of events may appear, they are not stringent enough to warrant any far-reaching conclusions. Yet on November 17, 1947, that is twelve days after the dream under review, and ten days after the session in which the waking incident with the knife was discussed, Mr. T. recounted a second incident involving a knife.

"Yesterday morning I was on the floor when some character walked in. He looked like a tramp, with a battered hat, dishevelled shirt and holes in his shoes; he looked fierce like a maniac. I knew him from before, he had come to our place three or four times before. I always watched him whether he was not out for stealing. But, as a rule, he bought something, stationery, pencils or so. This time he walked straight to the cutlery counter. I was just two counters away and saw that he picked up a large kitchen knife, four to five inches long, and said something to the girl at the counter though I could not hear what he was saying. At that he turned round towards me, looked at me and with a savage gesture brandished the knife towards his throat. I got very uncomfortable, in fact I ran downstairs to the basement. After a while I pulled myself together and went back to the girl at the cutlery counter. 'What happened to your boy friend?' I asked jokingly. 'Did he buy the knife?' The girl answered in the affirmative adding, still somewhat taken aback, 'He said, "When that guy bothers me I will cut his throat open." Then he paid and walked out with the paring knife.'"

The patient gave the account of this second incident hesitantly, with the same air of amazement as the first one, resorting to gesture to illustrate his narrative. A self-made man of average education, Mr. T. had no philosophical bent and was certainly not in the habit of introspection. The analytical experience was his first encounter with psychological problems of any depth. His common sense told him that, apart from their significance brought out in the analytical sessions, dreams could not possibly have any additional "occult" significance. I may also add that he had no inkling of my interest in parapsychology. Yet, despite his natural scepticism, the repetition of the knife incident, linked as it was with his dream, alarmed him. I repeated to him the interpretation of the dream and suggested that both the first and the second waking incident involving a knife may have been due to his increased awareness of such objects in his environment and, therefore, largely to his own state of mind. This explanation, I said to him, should dispose of any superstitious misrepresentations of his experience and would also account for the apparent duplicity of the cases described.

The question is whether it *really* does so? Looking once more into the record of the case we can tabulate the salient features of the dream and of the two waking incidents considered together in the following way:

Dream	*Waking Incidents*
5.11.47.	7.11.47 and 16.11.47.
A "guy" in the store who was after something; staging a hold-	A character coming into the store, selecting a large paring

Dream	*Waking Incidents*
up; brandishing a large "flip-open" knife. The dreamer runs away.	knife, threatens to cut open the patient's throat. The patient runs away.
The same "guy," sitting next to (alongside? opposite?) the dreamer in a much friendlier atmosphere.	A coloured man in the bus is seated by the side of the patient. The atmosphere is "friendly." (Patient is no longer frightened in the bus.)
He takes out a little pen-knife, an inch or so long, flips it open.	The coloured man takes out a penknife, an inch or so long. "It had the same little blade . . . like taken out of the dream." Flips it open.
The dreamer is relieved, thinks himself foolish to be afraid of the knife.	The coloured man takes out an apple, cuts it and starts eating it. Patient is relieved and thinks himself foolish to be afraid of the knife—and of travelling by bus or by underground.

It will be noted that in this table the relevant features of the two incidents are telescoped into one. They are used much in the same way as two complementary plates whose imprints are superimposed on one another to make a two-coloured print. Whether or not such a procedure is admissible will presently be discussed. The fact is that each incident contains a number of features which are suggestive of some correspondence. Yet the two incidents, considered jointly, seem to get very close indeed to the manifest content of the dream.

It will also be noted that in making up our table we disregarded the chronological order of the events listed on the right side, i.e. on the side listing the two waking incidents. The incident with the large knife actually occurred *after* the one featuring the pen-knife, while in the dream the patient was first pursued by a man brandishing a large "jack-knife"—to realize in the second part of the dream only that it was in fact but small and insignificant.

It might be objected that assembling our material in this manner is arbitrary; that comparing the contents of the dream with two separate happenings listed in the reverse order and occurring ten days apart runs counter to our rational way of thinking. So long as we confine our considerations exclusively to the rational plane this objection may indeed be justified. On the other hand, it goes without saying that once we enter into a serious discussion of the feasibility of such "intrinsically improbable" occurrences as precognitive dreams we must be prepared to forgo—at least for argument's sake—some of our familiar notions of the unalterable laws of temporal order, of the rigid and irreversible sequence of past, present, and future.

On accepting this working hypothesis, the correspondence of the two sets of events listed on the two sides of our table is striking enough. The two consecutive parts of the dream seem to duplicate the two real incidents described: the one culminating in the patient's flight from his pursuer, the other bringing home to the patient the futility of his fear of the pursuer's knife. The knife itself is represented as a large paring knife and as a small pocket-knife respectively. In fact, the small one seen in the incident appears to Mr. T. "like taken right out of the dream." Again, his fear and his subsequent sense of relief both in the dream and in the waking state are described by the patient in the identical words. Likewise, the pleasant atmosphere experienced in the second part of the dream may well be compared with the patient's feeling of relief on being able to sit alongside "the coloured fellow" cutting his apple in the bus without getting panicky.

These are the points of resemblance between the dream and the waking incidents. But it may also be well to cast a glance at the points of difference. In the dream the "guy" who was after the patient and who threatened him with a knife was a white man. Subsequently Mr. T. found himself engaged in a friendly conversation with the same man. Yet the fellow with the harmless little pen-knife who sat next to him in the bus was a Negro. They sat near each other, as in the dream, but they did not engage in any conversation. Further, the little knife was identical in both dream and the first waking event, but was described as a large paring knife in the second real incident, whilst it appeared as a big jack-knife in the first part of the dream.

There is a number of further features in both dream and

corresponding real events which, from the point of view presented here, may perhaps be regarded as irrelevant, but which might, nevertheless, be invoked as evidence against the assumed correspondence between the two series and the attending precognitive nature of the dream. Such minor points of difference are: The patient calls for the police in the dream but was not doing so in the waking incident. In the dream he feels threatened by his pursuer in some unspecific way, whilst in the real incident in the store his pursuer threatens him in a specific manner, brandishing the knife against his own throat.

One may well ask at this point: Is it legitimate to by-pass these points of difference as features of minor importance while the items listed in our table are credited with major importance? To decide this question we can take our lead from established principles of psychoanalytic practice. We know from experience that the manifest content of the dream may contain an infinite variety of items charged with varying shades of emotional significance. Thus we said that, from the analytical point of view, the large knife in the dream stands for a phallic symbol, representing a nodal point as it were, on which all the patient's pent-up fears and desires are focused. The *motif* of being chased by a male pursuer is of equal dynamic significance to the dreamer. The change to the harmless little knife in the second part of the dream, expressing as it does his changed attitude towards the homosexual menace, bears a slightly lesser emotional emphasis. Talking to the former pursuer in a much more friendly atmosphere reflects the same turn of the tide and may likewise be classed among the features of secondary importance. The setting in which this conversation takes place, and the words spoken, are not indicated by the dreamer. They are obviously of negligible importance.

It will be noted that the emphasis laid in our table on what we listed as the salient features of the dream amounts to an exact duplication of the distribution of emotional charge which is suggested by the familiar psychoanalytic approach. The table contains nearly all the relevant features which have to be considered in order to arrive at the latent meaning of the dream. If this is true it can be concluded that what we described in our table as a selective list of "important" items is in good keeping with the current practice of analytical dream interpretation and is, after all, fully justified.

The items that can thus be extracted from the manifest content of the dream are as follows: (1) a "guy" plans an aggressive action, (2) he brandishes a large knife in a menacing way, (3) the dreamer seeks to escape, (4) a change to a friendly setting occurs, (5) the dreamer and the previous pursuer sit near each other, (6) the latter has a much smaller knife in his hand, flips it open, showing a blade an inch or so long, (7) the dreamer is greatly relieved on seeing how foolish it was to be frightened of the knife.

On comparing these items with the two complementary sets of subsequent waking incidents we find the following features: (1) a man enters the store and behaves in a suspicious manner, (2) he purchases a large knife and threatens the patient with it, (3) the patient runs away, (4) in the previous incident the patient rides in a bus without being afraid to do so. There is an auspicious change in his phobic attitude. (5) The patient sits next to a "coloured fellow" who takes out a small knife, (6) the knife is exactly like the one seen in the dream. (7) The patient is greatly relieved at seeing that his supposed pursuer is harmless.

In this way there are seven clearly distinguishable features common to both sets of events upon which our argument of their telepathic—or precognitive—nature can be based. Although it is admittedly impossible to estimate the improbability of such incidents being due to chance alone, the odds against it would seem to be astronomical. In trying to assess these odds particular attention has to be paid to the unusual features contained in the waking events, both involving a knife under conditions which do not, as a rule, constitute a proper setting for such occurrences. A threat with a paring knife is a rather unusual happening in a big city department store. Equally out of place is the man cutting an apple and munching it quietly in a crowded bus.

A further objection which can be raised to the observation described here is doubt as to its factual evidence. In particular, it may be questioned whether the dream as well as the subsequent waking events were described in a correct fashion.

Against this should be held that I was fortunate enough to record the dream verbatim on the morning after the night it occurred whilst the patient reported the first waking incident within thirty minutes of its happening. The second incident, likewise, was caught red-handed, as it were, and put down in black and white hardly allowing for such a lapse of time as might tend to distort the patient's narrative.

There remains the objection of wilful deception by either the patient or the present writer. I have no reason to doubt the patient's veracity. In our analytical work he tried his best to give a candid account of himself, whether he spoke of his childhood experiences or of intimate details of his adult life. For him the incident in the store or in the bus was in no way different from other material that emerged in his free associations. Nor had he ever shown any evidence of ideas of reference or paranoid delusions. As far as the present writer is concerned, his verbatim recording of the incidents related by the patient was perhaps the result of his quick realization of their potential significance. As a rule I confine verbatim records to dreams reported by patients.

Whether or not these formal criteria are sufficient to establish the *prima facie* evidence of the present account must be left for the reader to decide.

What are the criteria contained in the evidence itself which can serve as the basis for a telepathic or precognitive evaluation of the dream? Obviously here, again, the final judgment rests with the psychological significance of the proposed interpretation. If it is true to say that the patient had been capable of catching a fleeting glance in his dream of a particular slice or segment of future events, the question arises: What, of all things, made him select just the two knife incidents as described above? We can perhaps obtain a clue in this direction from the psychodynamic appreciation of the material. I have already emphasized the phallic symbolism represented by the knife *motif* and hinted that the patient's unconscious fear of homosexual attack has to be considered as the main conflict underlying his neurosis. It is this fear which may have made him particularly prone to feeling threatened by "knives and knaves" wherever he came across them—in the past, in the present and in the future. In this respect he seems to be in the same boat as certain types of compulsion neurotics suffering from phobias of sharp or pointed objects.

Although this does not explain the subsequent emergence out of the conjurer's hat, as it were, of the two knife incidents in real life, it at least throws the peculiar *patterning* or *structuralization* of the patient's waking and dream experiences into sharper perspective. It will be noted that, irrespective of the problem of precognition, in both series special emphasis is attached to certain well-defined emotionally charged areas within the texture of the patient's dream and waking experience. This results in the impression that the items concerned seem to stick out, as it were, from the universe around him. They seem to be illuminated like an object picked out by a searchlight from the surrounding darkness. One could say that both dream and actuality share the characteristics of an emotional gradient, with highly charged emotional elements occupying the upper part of the gradient and gradually fading towards emotional indifference at the bottom. The dream, in duplicating this peculiar pattern or structuralization of the patient's waking experiences acts much in the same way as the creative artist who decides to select a few important features of a landscape or of a human subject for pictorial reproduction, leaving all that is immaterial or accidental out of the picture. In short, the dream behaves according to the principle of figure and ground formation as brought out by the configurationist school of psychology.

There are other psychodynamic considerations which call for comment if we are altogether prepared to take the precognitive aspects of the dream into serious consideration. After four months of analytical treatment the patient had remained quite incapable of filling in a large amnestic gap referring to events in his childhood between the ages of three and six. This amnestic gap persisted in the further course of the treatment and was never filled. Instead a profusion of oral and anal sadistic fantasies, intermingled with barely disguised incestuous wishes, dominated the picture during the months preceding the dream, testifying to the intensity of his early infantile conflict. Has this marked trend to neurotic repression set into motion Mr. T.'s frantic effort to turn away from the past, associated with the tendency to reach out in his dream, in a vicarious manner, as it were, into the future, picking its manifest content from the sunny, not from the seamy side of the time continuum? Or is it the patient's defence against the anal aspects of life in general that makes him shun everything and anything belonging to the "behind" both in the anatomical and the temporal sense, as suggested by Dr. Jule Eisenbud[33e] in the discussion of Mr. T.'s case? All this must remain a matter of speculation at the present moment. But here, again, more light can be thrown on the presumed precognitive aspect of the dream when considering the situation from my point of view at the time it occurred.

I was engaged in correcting the galley proofs of an article on telepathy. This had renewed my earlier interest in the puzzling problem of precognition. My interest received an added stimulus by a conversation with a friend—the same one, by the way, for whom I had prepared excerpts from the German literature on warts, with the result described in Chapter V. This time my friend recounted to me a precognitive dream of his own which occurred under unusually favourable conditions of observation. My attitude toward precognition, still undecided at that time, thus received at least a bias towards its serious consideration. Three days later Mr. T. produced the dream just described.

It will be recalled that much the same attitude of emotionally coloured expectation was found to be one of the predisposing factors in some of the telepathic occurrences discussed in previous chapters. The difference between them and the present case only lies in the fact that here, for once, the patient seemed to oblige with providing just that unfamiliar type of phenomenon which had so recently attracted my attention. This, however, seems to be the only way, if any, in which factors operating on my side had been reflected in Mr. T.'s dream. In any case there is nothing in its manifest content to suggest the presence of heteropsychic material originating directly from the therapist and woven into the texture of the patient's productions.

There is, however, another factor which may have played

an important part in the making of the dream. Here too, as in the previous cases, due allowance must be made for the patient's positive transference to the therapist at the time the dream occurred. The dream itself gives a clue in this direction when the dreamer hastens to call in the police to protect him from the homosexual aggressor. Clearly, the police is the therapist himself. This part of the dream reveals the growing sense of security which Mr. T. had acquired in the treatment situation. Earlier dreams had already indicated that he was ready to abandon his original ambivalent attitude towards the analyst. He ceased to regard him as a source of homosexual danger. His account of the friendly conversation with the former pursuer holding a ridiculously small knife in his hand points in the same direction. In fact, it was immediately following the account of the dream that the therapist felt that he should lay before the patient a full interpretation of the homosexual aspects of his unconscious conflict. He told him that he was apparently no longer afraid that men might accost him in the street, in the bus or in the underground and sought to allay his castration fears attached to sex in general. Mr. T. accepted this interpretation with all the signs of profound emotion, indicating that the message had struck home. The reader will recall that at the end of the session he was encouraged to take the first step toward overcoming his phobia. Two days later, for the first time since the start of the treatment, he actually came to his session all by himself, riding in a bus—and reported the first knife incident.

Quite obviously the dream itself had occurred at an important point of the therapy marking the turn of the tide of Mr. T.'s intrapsychic conflict. Whether or not this change was brought about by the insight achieved or was in itself an indication that the patient had become susceptible to the analyst's unverbalized therapeutic expectations in a telepathic way will be discussed at a later stage of our argument. The fact is that the emergence of the critical dream coincided in a striking way with the dramatic improvement of his condition.

Summing up, it can be stated that the peculiar—seemingly precognitive—aspect of the dream was occasioned by two different yet mutually reinforcing sets of circumstances: (1)

the therapeutic *rapport* or positive transference in the analytic situation had reached a critical point; (2) my interest in the matter of precognition had received an added stimulus by pertinent observations related to me by a friend. One could say that here, again, the dream had occurred at the exact intersection of two lines of force, as it were, that can be plotted within two overlapping emotional fields: the one pertaining to the patient, the other pertaining to the therapist.

Unfortunately this interpretation leaves the most puzzling problem presented by the dream still unaccounted for: its apparently precognitive nature.

It will be noted that in seeking to apply the familiar psychoanalytic concepts to its manifest content we proceeded from the more or less tacit presupposition that the bizarre temporal reversal and transposition of events which were reflected by the dream and later followed in its wake in two instalments were immaterial to the psychodynamic appraisal of the dream itself. We proceeded as though the subsequent waking incident could legitimately be dealt with in exactly the same way in which we are wont to consider residues from the days or weeks *preceding* the dream, as an important source of the raw material from which its manifest content is derived. There is indeed nothing to justify such a venture—except for the purely pragmatic consideration of its consistency with a revised and expanded scheme of dynamic psychiatry to which we have referred on previous pages.

It is interesting to note that, except for the lack of psychoanalytic orientation, J. W. Dunne, the author of *An Experiment with Time*,[31] has applied just this approach to our problem. He makes the point that precognitive dreams are much more frequent than even the most enthusiastic advocate of parapsychology would allow. Dreams, he submits, are basically derived from two equally important sources: from the past and from the future. Dreams have a Janus face. They look backward and forward at the same time. They are connected with both sides of the associational net, as it were, with one stretching back into the past and with one reaching out into the future. Yet since we usually confine our analysis to retrospective aspects only it is not surprising that the precognitive element escapes our attention. Dunne describes a number of dreams dreamt by himself and his associates to show that on closer examination past and future "resemblances" are blended in equal proportions in ordinary dreams. Proceeding from observations like these he arrives at a new concept of man's relationship to time and puts forward his ingenious theory of a Serial Universe, subject to what he describes as the infinite regress of time.

Dunne's theory of time has been subjected to scathing criticism by such authorities as Professor C. D. Broad[14], M. C. Cleugh[21] and others from a purely philosophical point of view. It therefore falls outside the scope of the present approach. But apart from shortcomings of a philosophical nature Dunne's theory has another deficiency: it is based on a wrong assumption. The occurrence of tagged, i.e. strictly identifiable precognitive elements in the dream undoubtedly is just as rare an occurrence as the intrusion of ordinary "tagged" telepathic experiences into the dream. This is why most observers who sought to duplicate Dunne's experiments have met with failure. Indeed it may well be that Dunne's extravagant claims have contributed much to discrediting the case for precognition in the eyes of the scientific world. The refutation of his philosophical and mathematical theories has added a *coup de grace* to his laborious investigations.

How, then, should we account for what, for lack of a better designation, was described as the puzzling precognitive aspect of the dream discussed here?

CHAPTER IX

Precognition and Self-Fulfilment

IN the previous chapter we proceeded with the discussion of Mr. T.'s dream as though its psychoanalytic interpretation in relation to his basic conflict and to his experiences, past, present, and future, were the only thing that mattered, and we glossed over the difficulties involved in its hypothetical precognitive implications. But there is no use denying the "intrinsic improbability" of such an assumption. Any theory allowing for the possibility of true foreknowledge of future events implies the possible reversal of the causal chain. That is, we are led to assume that although certain elements contained in the manifest content of a dream were only to take place at some future point of the time continuum, they are nevertheless capable of affecting the nervous system of the dreamer in such a way as to give rise to all the physical concomitants of his dream experience and to his subsequent verbal account of the dream a number of days prior to the actual occurrence of the events.

But is this unorthodox interpretation of Mr. T.'s dream really necessary? Is it the only alternative to our brushing it aside as a mere chance coincidence? Once we have succeeded in clearing our minds of the conventional clichés of our thinking there is indeed another interpretation which, if only for the sake of argument, has to be taken into consideration. One could look at such incidents the other way round, as it were, and ask the question: Is it possible that Mr. T., instead of anticipating, in some unaccountable way, future events in his dream, had rather been instrumental in their actual occurrence? This may appear as a much more easily defensible working hypothesis. Yet we will presently see that it requires a complicated set of auxiliary hypotheses, involving telepathy of a novel type: the assumption of direct telepathic influences affecting another person's actual behaviour and, beyond that, his social and physical environment at large.

Reversing our chain of reasoning in such a way, we would have to assume that it was the dreamer's own unconscious preoccupation with the threat of homosexual aggression which made him fear that the "wild man" in the store might walk straight to the cutlery counter, pick out a big paring knife, threaten to cut his throat, etc. Likewise, we would have to assume that it was the patient's need to allay his anxiety, provoked by the coloured man sitting by his side in the bus, which gave rise to the more comforting thought: "Well, the danger may not be so great after all; his knife is just a harmless pocket-knife, not an instrument to rape or castrate with, but to cut an apple into slices." If in both instances his opposite number did in actual fact behave as Mr. T. expected, this would then have to be attributed to telepathy in a broader sense, that is, to telepathy causing the percipient to act in a way determined by the agent's thought processes—instead of merely "picking" his brain in order to obtain information or to "read" his mind in terms of a more conservative conception of the telepathic process. Moreover, we would have to add to this dynamically reinforced notion of telepathy all the physical props and prerequisites that are needed for the staging of the incidents foreshadowed in the dream. The "suspicious character" would have to step into the store at the right time; he would have to have the money ready to pay for the knife; the coloured man would have had to make sure to have both his pen-knife and his apple handy before boarding the bus, and so on and so forth. This is certainly a rather strained and far-fetched hypothesis. Yet it may well seem more palatable to the sceptic than anything amounting to such a shocking departure from scientific reasoning as the assumption of true foreknowledge of future events. But is it?

It will be noted that our second and more conservative interpretation, seeking to avoid the devil of precognitive telepathy, only leads to the deep sea of virtually unlimited action at a distance and in all directions, that is, to a notion precariously reminiscent of the idea of telepathic magic held by primitive man.

This dilemma is, however, intrinsic to our problem. Any allowance made for the occurrence of action at a distance—mental or physical—is bound to upset our familiar concepts of time, space, and causality. Conversely, once we are prepared to take the knowledge of future events for granted we may be forced seriously to consider the possible reversal of the "irreversible" one-way course of causality. It is as though the admission of any irregularity in one category entailed a corresponding distortion in the others. Indeed, the very assumption of possible precognition seems to be interchangeable with the idea of something like a telepathically induced arrangement of future events.

This idea is tacitly implied in some of the timeless myths and legends which have been among the building stones of our contemporary Western culture. The Oedipus myth, this time-honoured standby of psychoanalytic theory, is a case in point. King Oedipus, seeking to escape the inevitable doom which was revealed to him by the Oracle, flees from Corinth, meets Laius of Thebes on the crossroads and murders him, unaware of the fact that he is thus fulfilling the prophecy that he would kill his father. Here, again, the precognitive interpretation of the myth can be replaced by the assumption that it was Oedipus's foreknowledge of his doom which had provoked the fateful dispute on the crossroads of Phocis in which Laius raised his hand against his son in order to be slain in the ensuing scuffle.

In a similar vein it could be asserted that it was Macbeth's unconscious desire to slay and to put himself into the place of Duncan, the fatherly king, to which the Weird Sisters responded in a telepathic way, inspiring their prophetic utterances and thereby setting in motion the chain of events which ultimately leads to the fulfilment of their prediction.

This formulation leads us back to more familiar ground. Professor C. D. Broad,[14] of Cambridge, in discussing the problem of precognition from the philosophical point of view, has pointed out that what can be termed irreducibly "pre-presentative" precognition has to be neatly distinguished from cases in which closer analysis would invalidate the claim of true foreknowledge. Thus apparent precognition may be suggested by an incident the foreknowledge of which is derived from deliberate rational inferences from past or present facts and the laws of nature. It may depend on experience of other persons, or on associations formed by previously repeated regularities of our own observation; on our knowledge of the habitual effects of our own or of other persons' actions; or on expectations which tend to bring about their own fulfilment.

In any case, whenever something like the telepathically induced acting out by other persons of the dreamer's own fears and expectations can be resorted to as an alternative hypothesis the argument in favour of precognition loses much of its cogency. Reverting to Mr. T. it could be argued with equal justification that the patient did not actually foresee the future in his dream. It may have been the dreamer himself who induced the "wild man" in the store, or his fellow passenger in the bus, to act out his own ideas, conscious or unconscious. In short, it was the residues of Mr. T.'s dream content that acted as a present stimulus determining overt behaviour of those involved in a telepathic way, *here* and *now*. In fact such cases of apparent precognition in dreams as were recently described by Montague Ullman,[133] Jule Eisenbud[33e] and Gotthard Booth[12] easily lend themselves to such a more conservative interpretation.

Observations of this type can be contrasted with dreams which are quite obviously apt to bring about their own fulfilments. Such cases were described by H. Zulliger[138] nearly twenty years ago. This is also illustrated by the following case. Mr. Z., a man of forty-three suffering from cancer phobia as an expression of his castration anxiety, reported the following dream: "I ran the blade of my razor through my thumb. I felt a sharp pain." The patient's associations led him to the image of a sabre-toothed tiger of which he had been afraid in his childhood and to a recent rash in his left inguinal region which had aggravated his castration fears. Three days later, Mr. Z. came to my office with a bandage on his left thumb. Still under the impression of the dream related during the previous session I asked for an explanation. "Oh, no," retorted the patient. "It was not a dream. The day before yesterday, while sharpening my razor, my finger slipped and that is how I cut my thumb."

He had completely forgotten the dream which anticipated his accident by twenty-four hours. It is interesting to note that another dream reported by the same patient, and described in Chapter VII, also deals with a future development: with the anticipated ending of his treatment. In effect it showed his readiness for termination and played an important part in determining future therapeutic action taken by the analyst.

What, then, is the difference between observations like these and Mr. T.'s apparently precognitive dream? Using the nomenclature which has well served its purpose in the discussion of telepathy in general one could say: whilst in Mr. Z.'s case apparent foreknowledge and subsequent fulfilment are confined to a chain of events mental and physical, pertaining to the *autopsychic* sphere (that is, to what may be called a closed operational system of a self-contained and isolated personality structure), the system we are dealing with in the case of Mr. T. is one in which the chain of events involved extended to the *heteropsychic* sphere, affecting two or more persons besides the dreamer. To put it in other words: when Mr. Z. dreams of having cut his thumb—and subsequently does so in actual fact—we must assume that his injury is the exclusive and purely private concern of Mr. Z.'s—in any case, one largely confined to his intrapsychic conflict. By contrast, Mr. T.'s two knife incidents, affecting as they did two more persons involved in the plot, have to be considered as "public." More generally speaking, they suggest that the problem of precognition cannot adequately be dealt with within our traditional scheme of thinking about personality as a closed and strictly isolated functional unit. It involves the concept of telepathy occurring within a vastly expanded operational system requiring at the same time a new approach to the age-old problems of time, space, and causality as the three principal modes or categories of our thinking.

It should be noted at this point in passing only that attempts at a theoretical appraisal of a vast group of experiments with extrasensory perception carried out in recent years have led to much the same problem. One of the more technical controversies in the field of experimental parapsychology revolves around the interpretation of test results in terms of either pure telepathy, or of what Dr. Rhine[103] describes as "precognitive clairvoyance." The theory of precognitive clairvoyance suggests that a percipient, instead of responding to the mental image existing in the agent's mind, may conceivably receive the extrasensory impression of the subsequent written record of the target "ahead of time." Another group of observations involving the so-called PK or psychokinetic effect, that is, an assumed mental action at a distance affecting the behaviour of falling dice, posed the question as to whether or not here, too, precognitive clairvoyance instead of PK was involved. Alternatively, as a matter of purely theoretical reasoning, the possibility could not entirely be ruled out that a psychokinetic effect, involving all the paraphernalia of an ESP experiment—including the method of randomization, of shuffling cards, of recording procedures, etc.—may ultimately be responsible for the semblance of precognition obtained by such experimenters as S. G. Soal and K. M. Goldney,[118] Whately Carington,[18] and Dr. Rhine himself.[103b] C. T. K. Chari,[20] in a recent Note on Precognition, recalls that the problem has puzzled psychical researchers for many years. He quotes several investigators favouring the theory of self-fulfilment—or PK—versus precognition.

Even though the present trend in parapsychology moves toward clear-cut experimental discrimination between these two types of *psi* phenomena, it is hard to escape the impression of their close interdependence—if not interchangeability. The individual incident seems to behave like a pebble thrown into a pond, with the concentric ripples caused by its impact affecting the three principal categories of our thinking simultaneously. It cannot be surprising that the world reflected by such a rippled surface seems to be oddly distorted—in what some may take to be a flagrant violation of the laws of optics and of nature at large. But it is needless to say that whatever irregularity is suggested by the occurrence of *psi* phenomena is due to the rigidity of our scientific frame of reference and not to the "irregularity" of the facts themselves. It cannot be denied that *psi* phenomena are in contradiction to our customary spatial and temporal concepts. But if this is true there is only one practical conclusion which can be drawn from this state of affairs: we must try to apprehend the occurrences within a new scientific frame of reference from which the signposts of time, space, and causality have been removed.*

This is admittedly a difficult venture, particularly so when we bear in mind that our whole perceptual world is essentially based on spatial and temporal concepts. Indeed what we described as the criterion of specificity, based on telepathic tracer effects, is nothing but the time and space structured surface appearance of a few "striking" telepathic incidents. In the last analysis it is the presence of such "tagged" elements, e.g. in the manifest content of a dream, which makes their scientific investigation possible.

The modicum of spatial and temporal organization which can be discerned in such elements should not, however, obscure the essentially metalogical, extratemporal, and extra-spatial character of *psi* functions. Or to be more specific: combining as they do the qualities of two different levels of human experience they are of an essentially *amphibious* nature.

Once we are ready to proceed from this, at bottom purely phenomenological description, the deck seems to be cleared for the closer examination of the observations reviewed in the preceding chapters from the psychodynamic point of view—regardless of their otherwise disturbing philosophical implications. Indeed, we have seen time and again that despite their apparently capricious, haphazard nature they are governed by the same laws which apply to the dream, to the neurotic symptom and to unconscious processes in general. In short, they are subject to established psychodynamic principles. We may recall Ruth's telepathic dream discussed in Chapter III,

* A. Schopenhauer, more than a hundred years ago, arrived at much the same conclusion. Taking his cue from his particular version of Kant's transcendental idealism; from a few striking observations of his own (one closely resembling the dynamics of the apparently precognitive dream described here); and from the flimsy evidence contained in the writings of Mesmer, Justinus Kerner and their forerunners in classical antiquity, he suggests that so-called somnambulistic phenomena stand outside the Kantian categories of Time, Space and Causality. In his view the barriers separating person from person belong to the world of mere appearances, and interaction unhampered by spatio-temporal obstacles is a matter of course in the realm of the "thing in itself" (*Parerga and Paralipomena*, Vol. 2, 1851). C. G. Jung, in his latest study *Naturerklärung und Psyche* (Rascher Verlag, Zurich, 1952), has apparently been profoundly influenced by Schopenhauer's philosophy.

expressing her desire to find shelter in the therapist's home and identifying him with a beloved father figure. Or we may call to mind the dream dreamt by Fred L. illustrating his wish to assume the analyst's (i.e. the father's) role in the therapeutic situation. The same considerations apply to Ronald's dream, featuring a problem both the dreamer and the therapist had in common and helping to allay the former's guilt feelings about its latent content. And there is, finally, Mr. T.'s purportedly precognitive dream expressing his castration fears and their dramatic resolution, accompanied by the telepathic self-fulfilment of the dream itself.

There is another important characteristic that has emerged from the psychodynamic evaluation of *psi* processes. We have seen that the individual incident is invariably charged with a more or less marked emotional emphasis. This is unmistakable in most spontaneous occurrences which were discussed in previous chapters. I hinted that in all these cases the distribution of *psi* elements coincides with dynamically laden areas in the interpersonal field. It is in this way that we arrive at the concept of an *emotional gradient* responsible for the field character peculiar to the *psi* level of functioning.

It will be noted that such a picture of the interpersonal field indeed cuts across the boundaries of isolated personality units and the spatial and temporal order of things in the physical world in general. The wavy patterns of varying shades and gradations of emotional tension which ripple the surface of our postulated field are obviously capable of spreading in all directions, unobstructed by obstacles of a physical nature. Nor do they seem to be blocked by any gaps between person and person which they may encounter. We can compare this state of affairs with the behaviour of iron filings spread out evenly on the surface of a chess-board. Here, too, the characteristic patterns brought about by a magnet held in the proximity of the board would in no way be deflected by the black and white squares painted on it. The iron filings obey the pull of the electromagnetic forces issuing from the poles of the magnet —regardless of other determinants visible to the human eye. In a similar vein we must assume that processes in the nature of telepathy and related phenomena are little affected by configurations pertaining to our familiar Newtonian universe.

Put in terms of the Gestalt psychologist one could say that the interpersonal field is patterned according to the principle of *figure* and *ground* arranged in such a way that the former would be immutable and lasting, like Plato's *Eternal Images* or Kant's *Thing In Itself*, while the latter is accidental and subject to change. Yet it would obviously be wrong to conceive of these primordial psychic configurations as purely static, congealed structures suspended in an extratemporal and extraspatial psychological field, comparable to the "Attic forms" in Keats' *Ode to a Grecian Urn*: "Forever panting and forever young." We have rather to think of them in terms of Jung's archetypal *motifs* of the collective unconscious, or of the semi-mythological instinctual drives populating the nether world of the Freudian id. They represent the foci from which the germinal forces of biological growth are derived. They may be the carriers of what Hans Driesch[29] has described as the *prospective potencies* of embryonic tissues in which each cell seems to know *ahead of time* the exact way and direction in which it is to evolve.

* * *

What, then, is the relevance of these considerations to the purportedly precognitive dream discussed here? They are intended to show that on the *psi* level no strict distinction has to be made between what Professor Broad[14] has termed "truly prepresentative precognition" or the actual foreknowledge of future events, as opposed to apparent foreknowledge of the future which is *per se* instrumental in bringing about its fulfilment and which can therefore best be described as *co-determining* or *predetermining* precognition. In any case it stands to reason that our attempts at making such a sharp distinction on the ego level are invariably defeated by the basically extratemporal and extraspatial nature of *psi* processes.

Two examples may illustrate the point. According to a truly prepresentative concept of precognition, we may visualize the past and the future as two consecutive pages of an open book. The passage which we are reading on the left page, spread out before us, is the present. It comprises a word or two—maybe a short sentence. It is largely identical with what William James described as the specious present and which H. F. Saltmarsh[109] has made the basis of his ingenious theory of precognition. The part of the page perused is the past. We know it has not ceased to exist following its perusal. The rest of the page and the next page to which we are presently to turn represent the future. This, too, exists in a way, yet outside our range of immediate awareness. As we go on reading we do not pay any heed as a rule to the text beyond the passage on which we focus our attention. This physiological sequence of events is disturbed on rare occasions only: when the reader catches a glimpse of a word or two on the next page, possessed of exceptional emotional significance to him, or when his expectation is keyed up in a particular way so as to perceive them outside their proper order and sequence.

Precognition, visualized in this way, would imply a strictly deterministic concept of the future. The words on the right page of the book are there regardless whether or not they are in our field of vision and no power on earth can change them. By contrast, the conception of predetermining or co-determining precognition presupposes the capacity of what we described as patterning or structuralization on the part of the perceiving subject. I intimated that this capacity is at bottom of the same nature as the tendency of our sensory function to carve shapes, configurations or Gestalten out of what William James[61] called the jointless continuity of space. To illustrate this capacity of the mind as applied to the shaping of things to come our spatialized comparison of the future with two consecutive pages of a book is, of course, insufficient. It may more appropriately be compared with the process of its writing or, better still, with the process of composing a symphonic work. The major outlines of his composition, so we are told, may stand out in the composer's mind from the outset. "Nor do I hear in my imagination the parts successively. But I hear them, as it were, all at once," says Wolfgang Amadeus Mozart in one of his letters. The composer Adrian Leverkuehn, the hero of Thomas Mann's *Dr. Faustus*, expresses the same idea when he says that the act of composing is performed twice, as it were. First, the composition is completed in one's imagination and secondly, it is put down with all details of its orchestration in black and white. Thomas Mann indicates at the same time that neither the successive parts of the symphony nor the phrases of which it is made up are strictly "predetermined." They are subject to change—within the limits of the rounded whole or configuration of the work, much in the same way as the behaviour of a piece of matter is inescapably determined by the laws of nature, while we learn from Heisenberg that a few solitary electrons may be at liberty to do as they please. Expressed in terms of Gestalt psychology one could say that the figure is foreordained while the ground is fortuitous. It will be recalled that this precisely has been the impression gained when we discussed the essential as against the non-essential features of our "precognitive" dream; and we also stressed that it was the essential features which seemed to anticipate the future incidents described, while the non-essential items failed to make their imprint on the things to come. All this goes far to show that the conception of pre-determining or co-determining precognition gives better justice to our case than what Broad described as truly prepresentative precognition, implying as it does the notion of a rigid and inescapable determinism.

But the question remains whether and how far such concepts as determinism, co-determinism or self-fulfilment, based as they are on the familiar laws of cause and effect, can be applied to the problem of precognition. Indeed, one may rightly ask whether such an approach to *psi* phenomena in general is altogether necessary. The chapters that follow will seek to provide an at least tentative answer to these questions. The extra-temporal, extra-spatial and a-causal aspects of *psi* will receive particular attention in Chapter XIX, discussing conceptual schemes and "frames of reference."

PART TWO

LEVELS OF FUNCTIONING

AN ATTEMPT AT A THEORY

If fibres are indeed all that is needed to do the trick, has not the earth pathways by which you and I are physically continuous, more than enough to do for our two minds what the brain fibres do for sounds and sights in a single mind? Must every higher means of unification between things be a literal brain fibre and go by that name?

FECHNER, *Zend Avesta*

CHAPTER X

The Ego, the Id, and Psi

THE reader who may have become unduly concerned at this point over some of the more unorthodox implications of our argument can derive consolation from the fact that the days of what might be called the classical school of psychology, based on a rigid Newtonian concept of the universe, were over long before the advent of modern relativistic physics. Such students of human and animal behaviour as J. F. Fries,[45] Herbert Spencer,[119] and William James[61] pointed out more than half a century ago that our perceptual world is largely determined by our mental organization, by our past experiences, and by our needs, wishes, and expectations. And they were all preceded by Francis Bacon's warning against the fallacies or *Idols of the Cave*, to say nothing of Shakespeare, who seemed to be well ahead of them all with the realization that "Time travels in diverse paces with diverse persons" and offered to tell "Who time ambles withal; who he trots withal; who time gallops withal and who he stands still withal."

Even Kant[67], the advocate of the *a priori* nature of time and space, granted that "the world of sense may be very different according to differences of sense perception in various world beholders" and considered the possibility that there exist living beings on other planets "whose time ideas may be different from our own." Ernst Mach[77] has formulated the concept of the relativity of physiological time and pointed out that little animals with fast metabolic rates may have a different experience of time than larger ones with a slower metabolic rate, pulse, and respiration. More recently Alexis Carrel,[19] Lecomte de Nouy,[89] Hudson Hoagland[55] and others afforded experimental observations to bear out this thesis. Needless to say, the new insight into the relativity of physiological time is equally applicable to the perception of physiological space. This point has been particularly emphasized by Mach, Spencer, and James. The biologist J. v. Uexkuell,[132] who made a special study of adaptative animal behaviour, asserted that every organism throughout life carries its private world with itself like an impenetrable shell. He holds that the same is true for the observer whose perceptual world, including as it does the awareness of his own body image, tends to seal him off completely from the universe. "His notions of time and space are encased in his private world. Consequently, there is no such thing as absolute space and time common to all human beings."

More recent contributions of experimental social psychology have confirmed this view. They supply ample illustrations of the structuring of our perceptual world and the relativity of our cognitive processes. Gardner Murphy,[86b] in his *An Historical Introduction to Modern Psychology*, quotes the work of M. Sherif[114] who, in a series of ingenious experiments, showed that a subject's way of perceiving is profoundly influenced by social, cultural, and anthropological determinants. The ingenious experiments of A. Ames[5] and his associates at the Institute for Associated Research in Hanover, New Hampshire, illustrate the same point. They show that the nature of our visual perceptions is largely determined by our past experiences, preconceived judgments, and expectations. W. H. Ittleson and F. P. Kilpatrick[60] conclude from findings like these that perception is never a "sure thing," never an absolute revelation of "what is." Gardner Murphy[86b] is, therefore, right in his demand that psychologists should pay more attention to their own mental make-up and to social, cultural, and economic vantage points from which they make their observations. He calls for the exact definition of the observer's position within what modern Gestalt psychologists call the psychological field. Failing this his statements would be meaningless, much in the same way as the physicist's pointer readings are in need of exact definition of his own position in respect to the frame of reference within which his observations are made.

Psychologically speaking, all observations registered by an observer are determined by the structure and functional characteristics of that particular level of personality which happens to react to—or to interact with—his total environment. The postulate of the relativity of our perceptual world is a partial acknowledgment of this state of affairs.

The theory of Gestalt psychology has sought to overcome the relativistic position by pointing out that the organization of sense data into meaningful wholes is an empirical fact, regardless of the perceiving subject's past experience, learning process, etc. But here, too, Koehler[70] has emphasized that sensory organization, in the last analysis, is an achievement of the nervous system, or of the "perceptual self," functioning as a whole.

Freudian analysis focuses attention on one particular level of the "self." While by no means neglecting structural aspects of the perceptual apparatus itself, it shows how our picture of reality may be distorted by instinctual drives, how the lawful operation of ego functions may be vitiated by the inchoate forces of the unconscious, subject to a different set of laws and anchored in more primitive, archaic levels of personality development.

Yet the psychoanalytic system of thought has stopped at this point. It has largely ignored the phenomena with which we have been concerned in the preceding chapters and still hesitates to advance its inquiry into *psi* levels.* This in spite of the fact that it possesses most of—though not all—the conceptual tools and technical prerequisites necessary for dealing with our problem. I propose to show in the following pages that what might be described as the *psi* level of functioning is closely related to the dynamics of the Freudian id[44d]—or, for that matter, to the dynamics of the Jungian Collective Unconscious. Thus our approach aims at the inclusion of a new dimension—or of a new and hitherto neglected level of functioning—into the picture of personality structure. What, then, are the charac-

* George Devereux' anthology, *Psychoanalysis and the Occult* (Internat. Univers. Press, 1953), published since this book has gone to press, marks an important new departure in the orthodox analytical position. It gives an comprehensive picture of the conflicting attitudes taken by leading psychoanalysts, including Freud himself. It also includes some of the recent papers quoted in my bibliography. By contrast, C. G. Jung's latest study, *Naturerklärung und Psyche* (Zurich, 1952), is an emphatic affirmation of the reality of *psi* phenomena and proposes a new theory of "synchronicity" for their explanation. It, too, reached the present writer after conclusion of this book.

teristics of the three principal functional levels which can be distinguished in this way?

THE EGO LEVEL OF FUNCTIONING

On this level of functioning the sky is blue, the sun shines warmly and the sensation produced by weights placed on our outstretched hand follows the Weber–Fechner law. More precisely, the elements of our sensory impressions are composed of and coalesce into organized wholes and result in patterns or configurations which, we learn from the Gestalt psychologists, are in turn derived from our own mental organization. Space is filled with matter and is impenetrable by matter outside the same portion of space. Time is an irreversible flow of events, mental and physical, and the laws of cause and effect—like Time and Space—are fundamental modes or categories of our perception. The picture of a world perceived in this way can best be described in terms of a three-dimensional frame of reference in which everything is connected in a lawful manner, in which two and two are four, in which parallel lines meet in infinity only and the shortest connection between two points is a straight line. Whatever happens in this frame of reference obeys a series of laws formulated by Newton and Galileo and later modified by the Maxwell–Faraday equations. In short, it is a world obeying the laws of Aristotelian logic, Euclidian geometry, Newtonian mechanics, and Kantian transcendentalistic psychology.

From the psychodynamic point of view, our actions on the ego level of functioning are—or should be—determined by what Freud described as the reality principle, based on the rational appreciation of all available data, including the anticipation of future happenings. They are controlled by our conscious volition and aim at self-preservation, at reducing inner tensions and at warding off excessive outer stimulation. In this conceptual scheme human personality is a strictly isolated and self-contained unit and interpersonal relationships are based on communication by means of expressive movements, language or other conventional systems of symbols. It holds that, whatever be the mode of their interaction, both the individual and the group are subject to the same laws of nature as apply to the universe at large, even though the appearance of purpose which enters the picture on the psychological plane may force us to combine the strictly mechanistic approach with an inquiry into goals and motivations. Although such an approach fails to give the answer to all our questions, we are confident that with the gradual extension of our knowledge we will gain an increasing understanding of both the world around us and of our own nature. In any case, such a picture of the world represents a well-rounded and logically coherent system and it is held that whatever flaws or irregularities are found in it are due to errors of judgment, optical illusions or to the outright mental derangement of its beholders.

In the early Christian era Satan was considered the villain in this play. He was made responsible for all interference with the strictly rational purpose and design of Creation. It was for Freud and his school to demonstrate the existence of deeper, "irrational" levels of our personality, to study their dynamics and to reveal their relevance to our rational, conscious behaviour. Yet to some of his followers—as well as to many of his opponents—the unconscious still is at bottom nothing but a caricature of the rational aspects of personality, a scientific derivative of the Evil in the Christian universe. In other words, viewed from the ego level of functioning or judged by the standards of the superego, the id appears in a distorted fashion, comparable to the distortion of outlying parts of the world in the Mercator projection of the globe.

Certainly this bare outline of the world viewed from the perspective of the ego is incomplete—and indeed cannot be otherwise. Our libraries are stocked with countless volumes devoted to just this aspect of the universe. In fact, pre-relativistic science has been nothing else than a study concerned with the accumulation of data viewed from the vantage point of the ego *here* and *now*.

THE ID LEVEL

I hinted that Freud's[44d] original description of the unconscious, later referred to as the id—is a picture of intellectual anarchy, of untrammelled and conflicting instinctual drives. The unconscious seems to defy the principle of cause and effect and to disregard the established rules of logic as they apply to the ego level: it is metalogical. On the id level the laws of contradiction are no longer valid. A statement may be both true and false. Love and hatred may stand for each other as heat can be converted into electricity and electricity into heat. Black may be white, the sacred may be wicked. Temporal order and sequence have lost their meaning; so have spatial relationships. The notions of past, present, and future are hopelessly jumbled. Distance is no longer an obstacle to action and action itself may be unlimited in scope and consequences when it is propelled by the driving power of the instinct.

It will be noted that an uninformed traveller catching a first glimpse of the strange rites and rituals of a primitive tribe may arrive at much the same conclusions. The stereotype picture of Barbarian ways of life as it existed in the Hellenic mind at the time of Herodotus; the crude misconceptions about the godless heathens of the medieval Christian era and our own tendency to misinterpret the mentalities of foreign nations illustrate the same point. Failure to conform with standards prevailing within a certain cultural group or intellectual climate leaves us bewildered and confused and is apt to provoke intellectual disapprobation or emotional repudiation. I pointed out in the previous chapters that *psi* phenomena, emerging as they do from a sphere outside our familiar orbit of experience, are subject to much the same attitudes of rejection.

But closer psychodynamic study of the unconscious soon revealed that the id, far from being as chaotic and irrational as it had appeared at the beginning, is governed by peculiar laws of its own. We may only recall the tendency to displacement, condensation, symbolic representation characteristic of the dream and the neurotic symptom. Again, what Freud described as the belief in magic and animism, in the omnipotence of thought, as the law of talion, and the like, are samples of archaic mental attitudes which have been preserved in the id like an antediluvian insect encased in a block of amber.

This more balanced picture of the unconscious was further

elaborated by Jung.[65] He sees in the unconscious the matrix from which all the creative forces of the mind have evolved and restricts the part played by repression in its development. Jung lays greater emphasis on the archetypal, hereditary, aspects of the unconscious. The archetypal images, common to all mankind, form the connecting link between modern man and the long line of his human and prehuman ancestors in the perspective of time. They are the ultimate source of religious experience, of creative inspiration and intuition in primitive man, in the child, and in the genius.

Whatever concept of the id will ultimately gain general recognition, Freud's original picture of the unconscious has undergone considerable change. The place of the untrammelled instinctual drives has been taken over by a well-balanced system of physiological regulations, independent of conscious volition, but subject to the control of deeper vegetative centres representing what Cannon called the Wisdom of the Body. This aspect of human personality—and of life in general—is not so much concerned with the physical environment with which the organism is confronted *here and now*, as with the regulation of its basic functions of growth, metabolism, and procreation. If the id has been accused of being under the unconditional sway of the pleasure principle and incapable of adjusting to and testing reality, it is now credited with a profound awareness of the biological needs of the species which is unattainable to reason "sicklied o'er with the pale cast of thought."

Like an imaginary traveller through space and time who may be at a loss to read the street map of his immediate neighbourhood but takes his bearings from the stars or from transcontinental mountain ranges and river beds, the id is guided by landmarks that have evolved in the course of phylogenetic development and is oriented towards goals inherent in the very process of evolution.

Indeed there is a vast body of experimental and clinical data referring to what has been described as the hyper-function of the unconscious. There are numerous reports of unusual feats of memory, of artistic creation, and even of mathematical reasoning in dreams, hypnosis, and in trance states. The well-known observations of unconscious time appreciation in post-hypnotic states and in hypnosis as described by Forel,[39] T. W. Mitchell,[82] M. Bramwell,[13] and many others are of particular interest in the present context.

In a series of experiments carried out by the present writer[32a] in his student days at the Neurological Department of the University of Prague, it was found that normal subjects who are utterly incapable of giving adequate estimates of the lapse of time in the waking state, are able to do so with striking accuracy during sleep or in deep hypnosis.

This is further corroborated by the observation that many persons are capable of waking up "on the dot" from ordinary sleep any time they set for themselves. This striking "alarm clock" effect has mistakenly been ascribed to the operation of *psi* factors. It is more probably connected with the inner rhythm and periodicity of autonomous nervous functioning and independent of the cognitive, intellectual aspects of cortical control. I have pointed out elsewhere[32b] that what may be described as the *unconscious time sense* may be found intact even in cases in which organic cerebral lesions have caused impairment of conscious temporal orientation.

One can thus distinguish between two basically different types of orientation in time: (1) cognitive time appreciation based on the intellectual appraisal of environmental factors (and consequently subject to the usual errors of judgment), and (2) the primitive time sense which is independent of data pertaining to the outside world and exclusively relies on impressions from within. "Errors" in the function of the primitive time sense seem to be due to irregularities on the physiological level. I have found that the unconscious appreciation of time was accelerated in patients suffering from hyperthyroid conditions which are known to be associated with an increased metabolic rate. I may mention by way of a footnote only that experiments indicating the existence of an unconscious time sense have also been carried out by R. Isenschmid,[59] and many others in ants, bees, and wasps. It was found that insects, when given thyroid extract to increase their metabolic rates, showed an acceleration of their temporal responses similar to that seen in hyperthyroid patients.

There is thus nothing mysterious about observations of this kind in both animals and human subjects. The only question that has puzzled workers up to our day is the way in which clues indicating the time that has elapsed, e.g. while the subject is asleep, are transmitted from the unconscious to the conscious level, from the id to the ego.

On reviewing the records of the observations described here from our present vantage point the answer is obvious. The unconscious time sense of all subjects participating in my own experiments functioned like clockwork on one condition only: when those involved were taking a spontaneous, emotionally charged interest in the experiments. In view of the youthful scientific fervour of both the experimenter and his associates at the time these tests were carried out they certainly met with this requirement. Many readers may have made similar observations of their own. They may have found their wish to wake up at an appointed time to be effective in the presence of strong emotional incentives only derived from a deeper level of their personality.

Despite differences there is, in this way, a far-reaching parallel between *psi* phenomena and the so-called hyper-functions of the unconscious discussed here. Both show the characteristics of two separate levels of functioning. Both are of an amphibious nature, as it were, and both are capable of breaking through the barriers separating one from the other under certain dynamically well-defined conditions only: when their occurrence happens to satisfy the deep-seated emotional needs of those involved. It is also interesting to note that our reactions to such occurrences may be similar in both cases. They may leave the naïve spectator with a feeling of superstitious awe or puzzled bewilderment over an apparent violation of the laws of nature. This also is the way in which the ancients are known to have responded to the sight of "tokens and portents" in the skies—to shooting stars or comets abandoning their predetermined orbits and passing through the atmosphere of the earth.

There is another point of resemblance between *psi* phenomena and id processes. It will be noted that most instances of hyperfunctions of the unconscious to which we referred in the present context are closely related to the state of hypnosis and sleep. It will also be recalled that this is equally true for virtually all instances of telepathy described in previous chapters. In fact, I pointed out that their occurrence is in part occasioned by what I described as a minus function, global or circumscribed, lasting or transient, and the tendency to its compensation. The primitive time sense which seems to be called to the fore when our conscious orientation in the world is in abeyance is in this way a striking counterpart of our potential susceptibility to telepathic influences under similar conditions.

The concept of a minus function as it is used here is, however, in need of qualification. Sleep, absent-mindedness or the state of passivity and relaxation which, we said, is conducive to the emergence of *psi* processes, implies a reduced level of functioning only when it is measured by the standards of our conscious orientation on the ego level. It is a minus function in relation to our classical three-dimensional frame of reference only. It may well be that both the *psi* and the id levels of functioning are biologically self-sufficient in their own right and by no means inferior to the ego level.

That only functioning on the ego level—that is on the level of our standard three-dimensional orbit of experience—is credited with positive survival value in our culture and that, consequently, other levels of functioning are subject to repression, social disapprobation or outright ostracism is another matter.

THE PSI LEVEL OF FUNCTIONING

Are we justified, after all, in drawing a strict demarcation line between the id and *psi*? Are they really to be considered as two separate levels of functioning, or is the distinction between them merely the result of our belated insight into *psi* coming, as it does, nearly half a century after Freud's pioneering advance into the Unconscious? Is *psi* a separate functional level in its own right, comparable to the ego and the id level, or is it better to be regarded as the functional equivalent of a sensory apparatus which the unconscious actually lacks but which, nevertheless, enables one unconscious to communicate in an extrasensory way, as it were, with another unconscious? It may well be that with our growing insight into the psychodynamics of *psi* the Freudian id will burst at its seams and be replaced by a psychological agency combining the functional characteristics of both Freud's primary process and *psi* functions. If so, our tentative discrimination between the two will have to be abandoned.

At the present stage we feel much like the seafarer who, on landing in a strange country, is unable to decide whether it is part of a huge continent from which he had originally embarked or a separate island—if not a whole new continent of its own. We are still engaged in studying local soil samples and minerals, in collecting what specimens of strange flowers and animals we can lay hands on, and in comparing them with the flora and fauna familiar to us from our previous experience.

Be that as it may, only a provisional picture of *psi* can be drawn on the basis of the available evidence and all attempted comparisons with the ego or id level of functioning cannot help but be largely conjectural. Our evidence is fragmentary for three reasons. First, because of our innate resistance to accepting the very possibility of *psi* phenomena. Secondly, because of the methodological difficulties attached to their scientific investigation. Thirdly, because of the nature of our mental organization, which, for biological reasons, seems to be ill-equipped for dealing with material of this kind. Nevertheless, the basic experimental data are here for everybody to examine and the spontaneous observations discussed in the present study should speak for themselves.

I indicated that the apparent disorganization of data pertaining to *psi* incidents is largely due to our habit of applying to them standards essentially derived from the ego level of functioning. However, on closer study of the phenomena we found that, viewed against the background of a hypothetical interpersonal field, they show a clearly discernible and consistent pattern. There are areas of high and low emotional tension—much in the same way as the gravitational field can be described as "strong" and "weak" in different regions, the emotionally charged areas being occupied by our repressed instinctual drives or by the perennial themes of love and hate, by the fear of genital mutilation or outright dissolution, and the urge for self-preservation and self-assertion.

Yet I also emphasized that on the *psi* level these areas of tension are no longer confined to individual "selves"; they cut across the boundary lines of strictly isolated and detached personality units, much in the same way as they transgress the conventional categories of time and space. Nor do we have to assume that there exists anything like empty psychological space between them. It is true that for the man in the street, adjusted as he is to a three-dimensional, tangible, and visible world, psychological "space" filled to the brim with thinly spread—or densely packed—lines of *psi* forces is difficult to conceive of. But he has the same difficulty in trying to conceive of an electro-magnetic or gravitational field whose existence is at best brought home to him by the Maxwell–Faraday or Einstein equations. He may feel hot or cold, or light or heavy in his head, as the case may be—but any direct perception of the "real thing" is even farther removed from him than *psi*.

We also found that whenever we are able to examine from the psychological point of view the circumstances of an occasional breakthrough of *psi* phenomena into the ego sphere it occurred precisely in areas of high emotional tension in the interpersonal field. In this respect it duplicates the conditions of an occasional breakthrough of id elements into the ego. That the presence of areas of high tension does not, however, suffice to lead to such a breakthrough will be discussed on a later page.

In keeping with their amphibious nature *psi* phenomena may occasionally emerge on the conscious plane with highly specific distinctive features attached to them. They may then attain a considerable degree of spatio-temporal organization, characteristic of the higher cognitive processes. This is what I described as the telepathic tracer effect—a feature superimposed on, if not altogether alien to, the telepathic process. In fact, we have seen that the higher the degree of organization and integration of the elements concerned, the more feeble is their ability to penetrate the barriers separating *psi* functions from conscious experience. Conversely, the lesser their degree of integration and intellectual organization the greater seems to be their capacity of filtering into another person's mind. Needless to say for the very same reason it may then be difficult or even impossible to ascertain their identity and their heteropsychic derivation.

Summing up, the term *psi* is applied in two different ways in the present study. First, to describe such various types of *psi* functions as telepathy, precognition, clairvoyance, and the like. Secondly, more generally speaking, to designate a particular part of psychic reality—and of the universe at large—which seems to be exempt from the familiar laws of nature, but is subject to established psychodynamic principles. As far as content is concerned a twofold patterning of *psi* processes can be discerned: in the horizontal they are structured according to the emotional charge of the elements concerned; in the vertical according to the degree of their complexity and spatio-temporal organization.

It is in view of this paradoxical combination of two different structural characteristics found in many *psi* incidents that I referred to their basically amphibious nature.

This condensed survey of the principal features of *psi* processes should suffice in the present context. Any attempt at further elaboration would be of merely speculative nature and would lead to the precarious proximity of certain prescientific, metaphysical or frankly mythological systems of thought. But here again it may be well to realize that on trying to give a coherent and sufficiently "rational" account of the id level of functioning we came up against much the same difficulties. *Psi* functions, like Freud's primary process, characteristic of the id, seem to fall outside our customary temporo-spatial logical scheme of thinking. They are essentially metalogical and we shall see in Chapter XIX that they call for a new scientific frame of reference for their proper appreciation.

CHAPTER XI

Levels of Functioning and Mental Metabolism

ALTHOUGH a patient suffering from gout, influenza or anxiety neurosis may be of a different opinion, modern clinical medicine and medical psychology have made it perfectly clear that structural lesion or impaired function of the organism is at bottom nothing else than a challenge for the organism to attain a new level of adjustment to changed conditions. Failure to do so leads to a breakdown of adaptative functions and ultimately to death. But successful adaptation, mental and physical, results in a virtually infinite number of variations on the theme of structural organization and inner experience. Perhaps the most striking variation of this kind is the schizophrenic disorder of personality with its bizarre distortion of thinking and feeling, tending toward gradual disintegration of the personality structure and loss of contact with reality.

In my earlier book[32] I have tried to show in some detail how the schizophrenic process abolishes the barriers between the ego and the non-ego and how this may be accomplished by the intrusion of heteropsychic elements into the patient's personality structure. The schizophrenic is threatened from two sides at the same time: by the uprush of autopsychic material derived from his own unconscious, and by the intrusion of heteropsychic material originating from the *psi* level.

Symptomatology in the advanced schizophrenic is thus made up of hallucinatory experiences, of projection of repressed autopsychic drives into the outer world, and of delusional reactions to his own sensitiveness to *psi*—especially to repressed hostility emanating from his social environment. It is at that stage that the patient's experience of time and space may show increasing evidence of distortion and disorganization, testifying to his gradual loss of contact with reality on the ego level and to his withdrawal to a timeless and spaceless world of his own. The following is a typical case in point.

A schizophrenic student aged twenty-one was suddenly seized by the feeling that his thoughts were racing at a tremendous speed. People, too, seemed to move and talk faster than usual. Their voices appeared loud, they would use obscene language and berate him. He would also notice that his awareness of things around him became much keener than before. At the same time the room would appear to be getting smaller, the walls closing in on him causing the sensation of pressure inside his chest. Or else he would note that everything, including his thoughts, moved at a snail's pace, whilst things in the outer world would grow larger and vague in their outlines. The walls of the room would recede and objects or people would appear far away from him. "It is like looking through a magnifying glass. There is plenty of time for everything and the voices I hear are less critical of me than before. I say to myself it is not worth bothering now. Everything has become indifferent to me and to the people around me."

Again, sometimes he felt that time moved at an irregular pace, as though the world would be switched from a slow to a faster gear, or the other way round. At the same time objects would look small or large, clear-cut or hazy, and his own body either very real and vivid, or flattened out, strange and remote.

Advanced schizophrenics may altogether lose their sense of reality or the experience of time and space. However, similar experiences, often connected with states of depersonalization, are well known in certain types of compulsion neurotics. They are frequently associated with peculiar sensations referred to the body image. Or else the feeling of loss of reality goes with the impression that time has come to a standstill, that the world has lost its quality of depth and all colours have turned grey and "watered down." Experiences like these are not confined, however, to psychotic or neurotic patients. It will be recalled that hypnotic experiments mentioned in the previous chapter showed occasional distortions of the time sense in terms of consistent acceleration or retardation in perfectly normal persons. Linn F. Cooper and M. H. Erikson[22] have found in more recent experiments that the time sense can be deliberately altered by hypnotic suggestion. Their subjects showed deviations of all conceivable types and degrees of subjective time experience, including experiences reminiscent of our schizophrenic patient.

Peculiar distortions of the time experience in organic cases were also reported by neurologists. O. Poetzl and H. Hoff[95] described two patients suffering from lesions in the thalamic and right parieto-occipital region who experienced spells of accelerated or slow-motion changes of the world time as well as illusions of objects moving in their surroundings.

In contrast to these quantitative changes involving the experience of time and space are cases showing gross disorganization and disintegration of spatio-temporal concepts. In the following observation of my own[32b] the injury affected both hemispheres in the parieto-occipital region. The patient, a medical student aged twenty-nine, was admitted to the Neurological Department of the University of Vienna with a self-inflicted penetrating gunshot wound of the head. The bullet had been removed by surgery but the patient was left with serious damage both to his personality and to his intellectual functions. His speech was halting; at times he was at a loss in finding the names of objects or persons, that is, he showed evidence of amnestic aphasia. His handwriting was impaired, showing slight agraphic disturbances. He was unable to perform the simplest calculations. He lost his way in the hospital ward and was confused about spatial relations. His drawings showed the same confusion of up and down, right and left. Fig. 7 shows an example of his drawings which he verbally described as follows: (*a*) a french window in his ward at the Neurologische Klinik in Vienna; (*b*) a face, *en face*; (*c*) the window latch; (*d*) a ship; and (*e*) a tree drawn upside down with the root at the top, the crown at the bottom, and the trunk in the middle.

The most striking feature in these reproductions is the utter disorganization of the material. It seems to be broken to pieces, jumbled like meat in a meat-loaf that has passed through a chopping machine. On a diagram illustrating a compass he indicated south and west in the wrong directions. In short, displacement, inversion, and gross deviations from the hori-

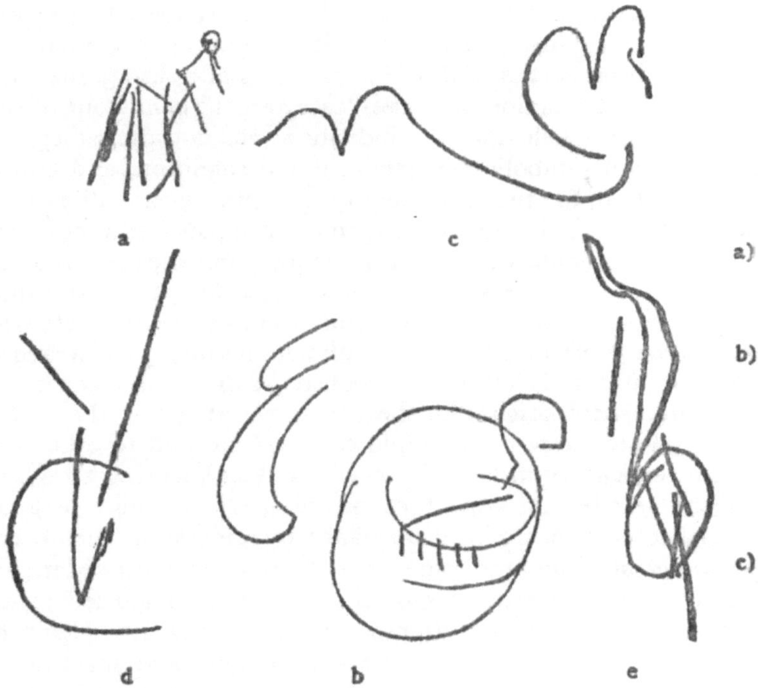

FIG. 7.—Drawings of the patient: (*a*) a french window; (*b*) a face, *en face*; (*c*) the window latch; (*d*) a ship; (*e*) a tree drawn upside down, with (*a*) the root, (*b*) the trunk; (*c*) the crown.

zontal were characteristic features of his spatial orientation and of his motor behaviour in space.

His mistakes in temporal orientation were of the same order. He could not tell how long he had been in the Neurological Department, nor the length of time he had spent waiting to be admitted to a surgical ward. He constantly confused data referring to his stay in Vienna and to his life prior to that in a small provincial town in Austria. *Before* and *after* in the temporal sense had lost their meaning to him much in the same way as spatial relationships. There was reason to believe that the patient's acalculia was likewise due to an inability to organize ideas in a consistent system of temporo-spatial relationships.

Since Gelb and Goldstein's[48] classical studies of the personalities of brain-injured persons it has become customary to describe disturbances of this kind in terms of a disorganization of the Gestalt function or of the "categorical" behaviour of the organism. It is held that the individual has not altogether lost his ability of symbolic expression, visual cognition, and motor co-ordination, but that his attempts at coping with reality move on a reduced level of functioning in a "shrunken" environment.

Viewing the behaviour of our patient against the conventional three (or four) dimensional frame of reference it appears that his principal disturbance affects just the hypothetical *categories* or *co-ordinates* of space and time. Although his injury has wrought havoc to all that is left of his responses on the level of conscious spatio-temporal orientation he can move about in the ward, he is able to carry on a simple conversation and to take care of the elementary needs of his everyday life. Focusing attention on the intellectual aspect of his disorder it could best be described in terms of a disturbance of orientation in the co-ordinates of space and time or as a *co-ordinative* disorder. To put it in other words: his incapacity can be regarded as an example of a patient's attempt at functioning on a level of experience from which the signposts of time and space have been removed through the existing organic pathology.

What, then, is the relevance of this observation to our problem? The parallel between the reduced level of functioning in our patient and the apparent structural disorganization characteristic of Freud's primary process as well as of *psi* functions as they present themselves within the orbit of our spatialized, Newtonian world, is obvious. We emphasized that telepathy, precognitive or otherwise, also seems to play havoc with existing temporal and spatial relationships. This spatial disorganization is well illustrated by Fig. 4 reproduced in Chapter VI. It will be recalled that it depicts the telepathic impression gained by Fred L. of my apartment with the adjoining terrace, etc. It also shows a radio aerial which I had installed on the terrace on the night the patient's telepathic dream occurred. Yet according to the patient his drawing represented a room in his mother's apartment in which he had fixed an electric cord, though he was puzzled over the drain-pipe that had "somehow" got into the picture. Nevertheless, despite these inconsistencies, Fred had received a fairly correct image of the terrace as well as of the way in which the aerial ("the electric cord") had been fastened to the fence on the left side—except for inverting the angle in which the last portion of the cord was turned.

Warcollier's book, *Mind to Mind*,[135] contains a number of illustrations bringing out the same point. Fig. 8 shows a rectangle enclosing five egg-shaped figures which were used as

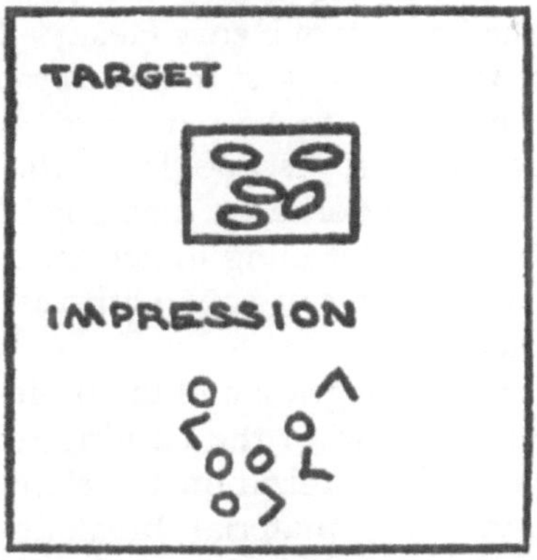

FIG. 8.—Showing the tendency to dissociation and disintegration of the telepathically received impression compared with the original drawing. (From Warcollier: *Mind to Mind*, Creative Age Press, New York, 1948.)

the target picture in the experiment. This target picture was reproduced by the percipient as five egg-shaped figures with four right angles scattered in space. Similar telepathic drawings have been published by Upton Sinclair,[116] Usher and Burt,[134] and many others. In all these instances a dispersion of elements occurs, as though an earthquake had caused a building to collapse, breaking it into pieces but leaving the bricks intact.

Comparing Warcollier's drawings with drawings prepared by the brain-injured patient described here, the similarity is unmistakable. It shows his inability to perceive and to reproduce the Gestalt of an organized visual impression. He can salvage only bits and pieces of the figure and makes it undistinguishable from the ground as conceived by the Gestalt psychologists.

This should not, however, obscure the far-reaching difference which exists between the two levels of functioning reviewed here. In the one case we are dealing with a gross impairment of cerebral structures involving vital adjustments of the organism as a whole. In the case of telepathic perception there is at best a transient minus function affecting cognitive processes but leaving the deeper resources of the organism untouched and indeed mobilizing them in such a way as to suggest once more the hypothesis of telepathy as an attempt at compensation on the *psi* level for an existing minus function. This has to be contrasted with the findings of Henry Head,[54] Kurt Goldstein,[51] and their associates which suggest that the brain-injured patient is left with but a modicum of patterned adjustment to his environment. He seeks to escape from the abstract to the concrete, from the symbolically meaningful to the immediately practical—from reasoning to action. This, they hold, is the only way in which he can cope with reality on a reduced level of functioning.

Summing up, the disintegration of the brain-injured patient's world of perception is due to the existing organic pathology, while the apparent disorganization of telepathic impressions, that is, of heteropsychic material breaking through to the standard level of experience, is due to the primary absence of temporal and spatial order on the *psi* level from which the material emerged. In fact, there exists a characteristic tendency on the cognitive level to complete and rearrange jumbled telepathic impressions in such a way that the disjointed fragments are built up again into new meaningful wholes. Warcollier[135] compared this biphasic process with the breaking down of a "psychic molecule," followed by the building up of its fragments into a new molecule.

On the biochemical level this process is known as the process of assimilation and dissimilation or as the anabolic and catabolic phase of metabolism which constitutes the two consecutive phases in which matter taken from the physical environment is first broken down into its constituent parts—atoms or smaller molecules—and subsequently built up again into molecules of greater complexity.

Heteropsychic material which passes through the barriers of

the ego seems to be subject to exactly the same biphasic process. It is first broken down to primitive, non-differentiated mental content and subsequently built up and reassembled again into ideational content of higher organization and complexity.

It should be noted that this distinction is not confined to *psi* functions alone. Freud[44e] expresses the same idea when he distinguishes between primary and secondary processes, the former pertaining to the unconscious, the latter to the conscious sphere. The primary process, Freud contends, has to be changed into secondary processes before it can make its appearance in consciousness. To put it in our words: such primitive material as a particular instinctual drive has to pass through a process of *anapsychic* organization before it can become part, e.g., of the manifest content of a dream. Interpretation of a dream then consists of a renewed *catapsychic* breakdown of the highly organized (and distorted) manifest content, revealing to the dreamer its primitive catapsychic core. This is illustrated by the chart on page 142 showing the biphasic nature of both mental and biochemical metabolism.

The one is thus the exact counterpart of the other, showing, once more, the basic unity of the life process. Psychologically speaking, ego and non-ego are separated by the same imperfect barriers as those separating the organism from its physical environment. Unless such foodstuffs as proteins, fats or carbohydrates are broken down into smaller molecules before passing through the mucous membranes of the digestive tract they may cause allergic or anaphylactic reactions. The same is true for the intrusion of heteropsychic material into the autopsychic sphere. It may either be broken down and assimilated by the ego, causing no reactions, or barely noticeable ones; or it may meet with resolute resistance and be altogether eliminated by the ego. Or else it may be felt as a threat to the ego and provoke anxiety, confusional states or delusional reactions. In any case, the massive influx of *psi* elements into the confines of the personality structure seems to be as incompatible with survival as is the breakdown of the physical barriers separating the ego from the outside world: "that way madness lies." An ego which has literally incorporated part of the outer world is bound to lose its identity. It may temporarily be inflated by

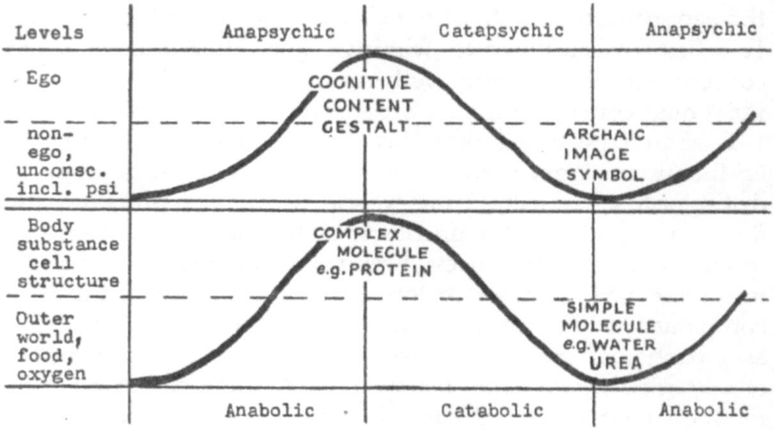

FIG. 9.—The two graphs show the tendency to biphasic change in metabolism, mental and physical. The top graph represents the biphasic transition of primitive, as yet non-differentiated, mental content into organized, cognitive material: a symbol becomes highly differentiated thought—e.g. when a percipient receives a disorganized, fragmentary image of the agent's mental content—and builds it up again into organized cognitive material. The bottom graph represents the biphasic process of assimilation and dissimilation on the biochemical level. Molecules of low organization taken up from the outside world are assimilated and built up into molecules of higher complexity (e.g. protein). They are broken down again and eliminated from the organism (e.g. as water or urea) and the cycle starts anew. The broken line in both graphs represents the barrier between ego and non-ego.

feelings of superhuman power and control—like in the paranoic's delusions of grandeur—or it may pass through the experience of communion with a divine agency—as in the raptures of the mystics and the saints—but adjustment to reality demands a detached and self-contained ego, isolated from the rest of the universe. The schizophrenic reaction type and the mystic way of life suggest that the evolutionary process has constantly been experimenting with various other modes of experience. But so far only adjustment to the familiar ego levels of functioning has proved to possess positive survival value in our culture.

CHAPTER XII

Empathy and Enkinesis—or How the Ego Reaches Out Beyond its Confines

---

THE revised and expanded picture of personality suggested by our approach opens up new vistas for our understanding of social interaction and intercommunication in both health and disease. Pre-Freudian psychology focused attention on conscious levels. Interpersonal relationships were thought to be determined by the spoken or written word, supplemented by gestures, intonations of voice and subtle reactions to unconscious expressive movements, facial expressions, and the like. Psychoanalysis brought the part played by non-verbal means of communication into sharper relief. It called attention to the way in which involuntary expressive acts—including psychosomatic symptoms—may reveal unconscious mental content. Freud specifically made allowance for the fact that one "unconscious" may be capable of communicating with another "unconscious" in the psychoanalytic situation, without, however, trying to explain the way in which such direct intercommunication is supposed to come about. The first part of this book contains ample evidence to demonstrate the part played by *psi* factors in this state of affairs. But it may be well to realize at this point that not all non-verbal communication is due to the operation of *psi* and that an important part of such communication can indeed be accounted for in terms of "subliminal" sensory perception and involuntary expressive acts to which we have just referred. In short, it occurs on a level closely related to the familiar sensory-motor functions of the ego.

But we shall presently see that there is a marginal area of ego functions which have attained a sufficient degree of differentiation to warrant separate consideration. They will be discussed here under the dual heading of empathy and its psychomotor counterpart, enkinesis.

Empathy is usually defined as the imaginative projection of our consciousness into another person. It presupposes a certain measure of *rapport* with the person with whom we are about to empathize, and it is this specific dynamic relationship, closely related to the process of identification, which seems to sharpen our perception of the many and varied manifestations of his personality upon which the empathic response is based. Viewed from a more behaviourist angle one could say that empathy arises from the actual sharing of various expressive acts, voluntary and involuntary, by two or more people. If this is so, we must realize that there is another, distinctly motor side to the empathic function. It is this motor or psychomotor aspect of empathy which is here described as enkinesis. Enkinesis can be defined as the imaginative projection of our consciousness into another person's motor or psychomotor behaviour resulting in the actual sharing of some of his motor, vasomotor or glandular processes. One could say empathy is projection guided by perception; enkinesis is introjected action guided by empathy. The two can thus be separated much in the same way as we distinguish afferent and efferent functions of the nervous system. Yet in doing so we must not forget that empathy and enkinesis are, nevertheless, nothing but the sensory and motor aspects of the identical process of social interaction occurring within a suitable dynamic context.

We have to realize, furthermore, that there is no sharp demarcation line betwen the two marginal functions of the ego discussed here and *psi* processes in the stricter sense. In fact, we shall presently see that there is a tendency in certain quarters to use such terms as empathy, intuition or extrasensory perception as interchangeable concepts or to speak of empathy or empathic linkage in a context in which reference to telepathy would be clearly called for.

It may be that it is this ill-defined, portmanteau use of the term which is responsible for the comparatively scant attention empathy has until recently received by both normal and abnormal psychology. First introduced into the field of art appreciation by Th. Lipps[74] in 1897, A. Adler[2a] emphasized its role in what he described as Gemeinschaftsgefuehl or community feeling, while C. G. Jung[65c] stressed its importance to the extravert type of personality. Some twenty years ago George H. Mead[80] and Charles H. Cooley[23] made the concept of empathy one of the basic principles of their system of social psychology. In a similar vein, H. A. Overstreet's[91] postulate of emotional maturity is based on the individual's ability to extend his range of identification and empathy from his family and next of kin to a wider group of his fellow men. In 1949 T. H. Cottrell and Rosalyn F. Dymond[24] published a series of experiments dealing with empathic responses in a group of subjects. They found that the ability to put oneself into somebody else's "psychological shoes" differs from subject to subject. They concluded that empathy played an important part in interpersonal dynamics and suggested that "shared patterns of attitudes and behaviour may constitute a concensus upon which rests the capacity of collectivities to function as integrated units."

In a recent clinical study of empathic responses in brain-injured persons Jan Frank[40] found a marked impairment of the empathic function going hand in hand with the loss of what Kurt Goldstein[51] described as the patient's categorical behaviour, while Frieda Fromm-Reichmann[47] called attention to an increase of empathic sensitivity in certain schizophrenics. Again, M. Levine,[73] discussing the therapist's approach to his patient, calls attention to the part played by the empathic element involved in their relationship. But among modern psychologists and psychiatrists it is perhaps H. S. Sullivan[125] who places the greatest emphasis upon empathy as an important link in interpersonal relationships. Sullivan attributed the peculiar emotional linkage that exists between mother and child to the operation of this factor and called attention to the fact that evidence of empathic linkage is unmistakable "long before there are signs of understanding of emotional expression or verbal communication between them." In Sullivan's view this feature of the infant-mother configuration is of great importance for an understanding of the acculturation or cultural conditioning of the human race. He holds that "both approval and disapproval of his performance is felt by the child through the same empathic linkage which has been so conspicuous in infancy."

Much less attention has been paid to what I described as *enkinesis* or the psychomotor counterpart of the empathic function, that is, to the motor aspects of "shared patterns of attitudes and behaviour" studied by Cottrell and Dymond. A first, purely phenomenological, approach to this aspect of our problem can dispense with reference to laboratory investigations. The part played by enkinesis becomes immediately obvious when we observe little Tommy sitting dreamily on his chamber pot whilst his mother, marshalling all her skills of dramatization, visual and auditory, is trying hard to induce him to do what nice babies are expected to do in his situation. At a later stage she will intently watch his first playful attempts at forming words, with her speech organs set to perform the task for him, with her facial muscles joining in and reflecting the emotions she and her offspring share between themselves and are about to express. Later still, when he is about to learn the use of knife and fork or the handling of simple tools and materials, she will eagerly follow each step of his performance and participate in it as if it were her own. She may tend to function vicariously on his behalf.

His teacher at school is less likely to get involved in the process of instruction with equal zeal. But Tommy himself, while watching a boxing match, will furiously clinch his fist with each blow his idol is about to land. His arm will bend into a protective arch to help him ward off an unexpected uppercut and he will jump off his seat yelling desperate shouts of caution and encouragement to the champion down on his knees.

His father, in turn, when giving him a chance to drive the family car, will contract each muscle of his right leg to make sure Tommy puts on the brake in time—if he does not altogether get tied up in knots at a dangerous intersection. He will then find out that backseat driving may be far more trying and exhausting than driving himself.

Despite the importance of the part played by enkinesis in

interpersonal relationships, experimental confirmation of its operation is still lacking. An interesting series of tests dealing with the telepathic factor involved in the process, using painful electric stimuli, was, however, attempted at the American Society for Psychical Research (D. Kahn and U. R. Neisser[66]). A series of clinical experiments carried out by Renold and his co-workers[102] may also be mentioned in this connection. Their studies are concerned with the effects of physical and emotional stress upon the circulating eosinophil levels in participants in a strenuous rowing contest. They found that while the members of the crew showed the characteristic reactions of the adrenal cortex to physical and emotional stress, the coxswains and coach of the crew had an eosinophil response largely comparable to that of the oarsmen themselves. No such reaction could be ascertained during the training period of the crews. Observations of this type, although primarily focusing upon clinical and physiological aspects, show the extent to which imaginative sharing and projection may affect the functioning of deeper, vegetative levels of the personality.

In these circumstances a variety of pathological deviations and distortions of the underlying attitudes, involving the psychosomatic sphere, can be expected. The anecdote of the German opera fan who sat through a three hours' performance of Richard Wagner's *Siegfried* and returned home suffering from a bad case of psychosomatic laryngitis is a case in point. The story suggests that even in the absence of tangible psychosomatic disturbance enkinetic sharing by one person of another person's motor or psychomotor attitudes may ultimately be accompanied by marked organic changes in the latter. In other cases it may fall short of tangible somatic pathology but may result in enkinetic fatigue, affecting a person's muscular or vegetative system—or his personality as a whole. Generally speaking, enkinetic fatigue may develop as the result of fruitless but persistent efforts to force motor or psychomotor behaviour patterns of our own upon persons (or things) in our environment.

An actual clinical example is the case of a woman of thirty-five, suffering from compulsion neurosis, who used to arrive in my office in a state of exhaustion whenever she had to take the bus. Afraid to be late for her appointment she would frantically try to make the bus driver go through every red light that stopped him on his way. Her magic did not work on the driver but her enkinetic efforts resulted in her breaking out in cold sweat and in stiff muscles on the following day. Many examples of sympathetic magic studied by Frazer[42] as well as their neurotic counterparts described by Freud[44f] follow essentially the same pattern.

The tendency to empathic and enkinetic sharing on the ritualistic plane is illustrated by the primitive custom of the *couvade*. The custom requires the father to take to his bed during his wife's confinement and to enact her groans and bodily labours in mock pain. Although it has no counterpart in Western civilization many a man fathering a child in our society will undoubtedly sympathize with the ordeal of enkinetic fatigue his primitive colleagues must endure in the performance of their ritualistic observances. There are countless reports of superstitious beliefs and practices in ancient times and in pre-literate people in our days based on the same principle, from the crossing of our fingers when thinking of a friend in distress to the magic ritual of the Hottentot woman who has to splash water on the ground while her husband is on a hunting trip lest he meet with disaster.

* * *

I hinted that, despite our distinction between the dual function of empathy and enkinesis on the one hand and *psi* processes on the other, strict discrimination between the two is rarely possible in actual life. Crossing our fingers for the benefit of an absent friend is certainly nothing but an ineffective gesture and there is just as little reason to believe that the labour pains of an African native mother will be eased by her husband's diligent observance of the rites of *couvade*. Again, it must remain an open question whether and how far little Tommy is likely to be helped by his mother's enkinetic participation in his performances on the chamber pot, while not even his father is likely to expect that his antics as an anxious backseat driver are apt to enhance the security of his ride.

But there is a number of observations in the literature of

parapsychology which indicate that empathic and enkinetic attitudes as described here may occasionally be at the very roots of telepathy observed in an experimental situation, even though the experimenter himself may be largely unaware of their operation.

In previous publications[32c, d] I described in some detail a case which illustrates this point. Ilga K. was a feeble-minded Lithuanian girl, aged nine years, who was suffering from mental deficiency superimposed on a marked reading disability or word blindness. Yet Ilga attracted the attention of her teachers and of the medical profession by her unusual ability to "read" despite her defect when her mother, situated in another room, or separated from her by a curtain, gazed silently at a sentence printed in a book, reading it to herself. Ilga's case, first published in detail by Ferdinand von Neureiter[88] in 1935, provoked considerable controversy among experts.

Two years later, Dr. Hans Bender,[8] now of the Psychological Laboratory of the University of Freiburg, reported on the findings of a commission delegated to repeat the Neureiter investigations under more rigid experimental conditions. The commission stated that most of the phenomena observed were of an auditory nature due to "involuntary whispering" by Ilga's mother though they did not deny that paranormal, i.e. telepathic, factors played a part, "at least episodically." Bender himself pointed out that purely auditory reactions on the part of the child had to be ruled out in those experiments which were carried out in the strict seclusion of a soundproof chamber in the Riga broadcasting station. But he makes a casual remark in his paper which calls for comment. Bender complains that in trying to duplicate the original Neureiter tests Mrs. K. could not resist encouraging the child with exclamations such as "Ilga think! Say it right!" or "Now go on!" etc.

He goes on to describe how the child recited the words read by her mother in syllables in a monotonous tone of voice, often impatiently, while "the lips of the woman who was of the excitable motor type and difficult to manage, were moving simultaneously with the child's utterances." But while this was going on no sound could be heard, and he adds specifically, "In one case the transmission of the word *saulite* (little sun) occurred so quickly that the mother had no chance of interfering."

To ensure objective observation simultaneous moving pictures and dictaphone records were made of both Ilga and her mother during the experiment. They confirmed that although Mrs. K. sought to help Ilga's performance by audible aids, some of the tests succeeded without real whispering on her part. They also confirmed that, as a general rule, "Ilga's mother moved her lips simultaneously with Ilga's answers."

Bender quotes a few more isolated observations which tended to invalidate the theory of auditory hyperesthesia, sensitiveness to involuntary whispering, or the like. They were largely duplications of Neureiter's earlier experiments. Nevertheless, another commission consisting of Latvian experts came to a negative conclusion.[8] They pointed out that, "Ilga K. does not actually read thoughts but merely reproduces, without generally comprehending their significance, sound-groups which, at least when her mother is sending, are formed in the motor organs of speech. The phenomenon seems to be a kind of mechanical imitation."

These brief excerpts from Neureiter's book and from the Bender report should suffice in the present connection. They indicate, first, that some, if not all, the phenomena described cannot possibly be explained away by resorting to the theory of mechanical imitation or sensory hyperesthesia alone. Secondly, they show that there was a striking *simultaneity* between Mrs. K.'s attempts to function vicariously on behalf of her mentally defective child and between Ilga's apparent response to what amounts to her mother's enkinetic attitude.

Unfortunately this significant correspondence does not seem to have aroused the curiosity of the experts. Failing to make allowance for the possible telepathic effect of Mrs. K.'s tendency to vicarious functioning they tried their best to suppress her uncontrolled behaviour as an undesirable source of error in the experiment. Yet their observations leave no doubt that although sensory clues were involved in some of Ilga's responses she performed equally well "without the aid of sensory channels" in others.

This should not be surprising if we realize that telepathy

may at bottom be derived from motivations which, on the ego level, manifest themselves as the tendency to vicarious functioning or enkinesis. We also emphasized that telepathy and subtle responses to sensory clues perceived on the ego level must by no means be considered as mutually exclusive. Bender's observations show in effect that the former may be a potential by-product of the latter. There is thus nothing "irregular" about the fact that some of Ilga's verbal responses occurred simultaneously with her mother's vocal or subvocal whispering. They only indicate that the child, while functioning as a telepathic percipient, behaved as though her mother's neuro-muscular innervations or enkinetic attitudes were in virtual control of her own vocal apparatus. She responded like a hypnotized subject to the hypnotist—with some of his commands getting through to the subject on the *psi* level.

The part played by enkinesis or the attempt at vicarious functioning is also illustrated by the following observation, to which I have already briefly referred in Chapter II. In 1938, Dr. R. M. Drake,[28] of Wesleyan College, Georgia, published the case of little Bo, a mentally retarded boy of eleven. Because of his poor school work his mother coached him at home. On this occasion she thought she discovered that Bo could spontaneously tell her words or numbers which she had not overtly expressed. "For a while he was thought to be a lightning calculator because no matter what the row of figures given he would immediately give the answer, provided it was in the mother's mind, but he could do absolutely nothing if left alone." One of Dr. Drake's students who had referred the child to him put it as follows: "The child cannot read unless someone is at his side looking on his book. He reads well then, but when left alone, he cannot read."

Bo had an IQ of 55 on the Stanford Binet Scale (Revision 1915). He was restless, distractable, and had a history of cerebral birth injury which accounted for his retardation. He showed a tendency to perseveration and verbigeration, could do second-grade work only, and was unable to draw a square or to repeat one of the sentences at age six contained in the Binet scale.

Dr. Drake devised a variety of additional tests to investigate

Bo's unusual abilities. He wrote down a series of numbers which were looked at by the mother and were to be called by the boy without seeing them. He made the mother read silently from a book entirely new to her and found the boy able to "repeat a large majority of the words, all the time paying no attention to his mother." Dr. Drake watched her lips carefully for incipient movements and listened for unusual verbal clues but could not detect any.

It is, however, interesting to note that here, again, as in the case of Ilga K., the mother was most eager to bring out the unusual abilities of her offspring. In the test situation she incessantly prodded the child, demanding better performance. Only with difficulty could she be restrained from butting into the experiment with remarks like "What is the next letter?" or "What is the next number?", frequently adding Bo's nickname as an additional stimulus. On one occasion she grabbed a stick to whip the boy with the result of improving his responses for a short period.

The most convincing evidence of Bo's paranormal abilities was afforded by a series of ESP tests of the Duke type extending over several months with the mother acting as the agent and Bo as the percipient. After overcoming initial difficulties due to his low intelligence, on March 6, 1937, the boy gave an average of 21 correct hits per run (as against the chance expectation of 5 correct hits) in a total of 14 runs performed on that day. One of the runs was "perfect"—that is, he guessed correctly all 25 cards of the Zener pack.

Most of these tests were carried out under so-called telepathic conditions, with the child blindfold and out of hearing of his mother, thus ruling out the possibility of auditory clues. Details of the experiment must be gathered from the original paper. I may only mention that Drake carefully ruled out all conceivable sources of fraud, collusion, clerical error, etc. He arrived at the conclusion that, using verbal signals given by the mother, and with the child functioning as a percipient, he indeed showed abilities which could best be accounted for by the telepathy hypothesis.

The parallel with the previous case is obvious, Dr. Drake's observations having the additional advantage of supporting his spontaneous evidence by exact statistical experiments. Taking them at their face value, the two observations suggest that in both children what we described as an existing minus function paved the way for a telepathic ability which amounted to a partial compensation of the prevailing defect. Yet, on paying closer attention to the attitude of the respective mothers, we have to amplify this hypothesis with the assumption that in both instances the compensation effect achieved was aided by their compelling need to make up for the social and biological shortcoming of their children. Our original formulation of a postulated minus function as an important predisposing factor of telepathic sensitiveness on the receiving end has thus to be supplemented by the part played by the *agent's tendency to enkinesis or vicarious functioning*.

Much less can be learned from the examples discussed here about the telepathic factors involved in the process of empathy. Describing Ilga's or Bo's reactions in terms of empathic response to their mothers' behaviour would unnecessarily stretch the meaning of the term. Both children were obviously far from trying to get into the "psychological shoes" of their respective mothers. Their telepathic susceptibility seemed to specialize, as it were, in heteropsychic awareness of such items as geometrical figures, spoken or written words or entire sentences—whatever be the reason for this selective effect. Such an effect indicates that telepathy has occurred "somewhere along the line" even though the elements tagged as telepathic may be of comparatively little dynamic significance to those involved. On the other hand, in the absence of tracer elements, the telepathic nature of material endowed with much higher dynamic significance may be difficult or even impossible to prove. Tracer effects are like driftwood carried by a stream. They show the direction of the current but are not identical with the current itself.

If empathy and enkinesis are the major tributaries of the stream only a small portion of its energies is transformed into what can readily be identified as *psi* functions. As a general rule, interpersonal relationships are sustained by the subtle interplay of both sensory-motor activities, empathy and enkinesis, and their extension into the heteropsychic sphere as indicated by such occasional experimental findings as those reported in the cases of Ilga K. and little Bo. In effect, the dual functions of empathy and enkinesis seem to occupy an intermediary position between familiar functions of the ego on the one hand and *psi* processes on the other. They form the connecting link between the ego level of functioning and *psi* levels.

CHAPTER XIII

Telepathy and the Child-Parent Relationship

THE two illustrative cases discussed in the preceding chapter were chosen to demonstrate the telepathic factor which is involved in two major aspects of interpersonal relationships: in empathy and enkinesis. I emphasized that it may not always be possible to decide whether or not a certain behaviour pattern is determined wholly or in part by subliminal sensory impressions, empathy or *psi*. But I also hinted that once the very possibility of *psi* has been admitted to our frame of reference the operation of telepathy has to be weighed as an alternative to such purely descriptive concepts as emotional contagion, empathic response, intuition, or the like.

Yet regardless of the nomenclature used we have to realize that it is from the coalescence of the vast mass of external stimuli impinging on our sense organs, of proprioceptive messages reaching us from the autopsychic sphere as well as from barely perceptible influences emerging from the *psi* level that the panoramic view of the world as we see it is composed. This is, of course, only another way of saying that human behaviour is basically determined by the integration and autopsychic organization of stimuli reaching the individual on the ego, the id, and the *psi* level.

This is indeed a logical conclusion from our preceding discussion but it has now to be tested against the broader background of interpersonal relationships in general. Our two examples illustrating *psi* factors involved in what amounts to a neurotically distorted child-parent relationship are cases in point. But they undoubtedly are exceptional cases due to the operation of such telepathic tracer effects as can rarely be seen in everyday life. Indeed, owing to the extraordinary circumstances in which they were observed they focus attention on artefacts. They must not, therefore, lead to the unwarranted assumption that similar tracer effects might be detected at the roots of the child-parent relationship in general. We must realize that this relationship is based on the sharing of much more elementary patterns of behaviour which have very little to do with highly structured ideational content, cognitive material, or the like. This, incidentally, is the reason why the telepathic factor involved has so far largely escaped the attention of the experts—with the result that they found it possible to explain most observations referring to the infantile and preschool period in terms of the accepted behaviourist or psychoanalytic theories. Specifically it has been assumed that the child is sensitive to his mother's facial expressions, to her tone of voice, to the way she is holding him in her arms, etc. In any case, reference to factors operating on the *psi* level is regarded as both unfounded and unnecessary.

A good example of this approach is a recent study by R. Spitz and K. M. Wolf[121] of 170 children observed during the first year of life. The authors describe a group of disturbed "faeces eating" or coprophagic infants whose mothers were depressed or melancholic. Their personality structure was in sharp contrast to the mothers of children who exhibited a tendency to rocking or to excessive genital play, but no coprophilia. Spitz and Wolf advance the hypothesis that the infants indulging in coprophagia and faecal play reflected in some way the unconscious tendencies of their mothers directed toward oral incorporation which Freud[44g] and Abraham[1] have shown to be a basic characteristic of personality structure in depressive patients.

They support this assumption with impressive figures and conclude that mother and child, during the infantile period, have to be regarded as a functional unit, as a "mother-child dual." During this period "most of the infant's functions take place in closest concomittance and interaction with the mother's actions and attitudes." Seeking to avoid reference to identification "which implies a specific mechanism" they speak of a virtual identity of the two due to a lack of differentiation between ego and environment. To this they add that "in this period conscious and unconscious, ego and id are not yet delimited in the infant" so that it is "easy to imagine the infant enacting unconscious attitudes of the mother."

Yet the question is in what way we must assume the infant to be capable of doing all that is implied by such "enacting." Dr. Spitz indicates that in some cases the "devouring oral attitudes" of the mothers were perceptible enough to be observed. But in other cases they were not. Have we to assume that the infants, in these cases, were able to make an unconscious psychoanalytical appraisal of their respective mothers' repressed complexes in a way which would give highest credit to Freud's and Abrahams's pioneering investigations?

Flanders Dunbar[30] attributes observations of this kind to emotional contagion between mother and child. In one of her cases the baby's mother had to be absent during the day and asked her aunt to give the child her noon feeding once a week. One day she noticed that all of a sudden her baby had developed an aversion to liver soup. She saw her making faces and spitting it out while her aunt murmured soothingly, "Now, Mary, just one more spoonful of this nice liver soup."

It was all commonplace, Dr. Dunbar goes on to say, but the mother thought her relative's expression was one of disgust, not so much with the baby's behaviour as with the baby's food. In fact she found out soon that the good lady had herself a violent aversion to the eating of the "insides of animals." Much the same thing happened when the child was given egg yolk prepared in a way which did not agree with the aunt's taste.

Dr. Melitta Sperling[120a] has reported a number of striking observations suggesting the ability of small children to react to the impact of the unconscious of their mothers in a manner which is difficult to account for in terms of the customary behaviourist scheme. One of her patients, Barbara, aged four, seemed to react to her mother's unconscious hostility in a manner "characterized by ambivalence and open sadistic attitudes with an increase of sadism and narcissism accompanied by an unconscious obedience almost as though she had to do what she felt her mother unconsciously wanted her to do." One day when the mother admonished her to be careful and not to fall on crossing a slippery street Barbara's reaction was, "Please don't tell me this or I will have to fall." Her mother's mention of the possibility of falling was to Barbara a suggestion or rather a command to fall. "She reacted to her mother's unconscious wish that she fall and not to the countercathexis in the form of a concern about her falling."

In another case the child seemed to respond to her mother's unconscious more in terms of sharing than in terms of resistance to the latter's unconscious attitudes. Ann, a girl of four, daughter of an obsessive compulsive mother, suffered from a severe phobia, vomiting, and abdominal cramps. Greatly improved through play analysis she had lost most of her symptoms. Yet Dr. Sperling reports that one day Ann suddenly relapsed into the old symptoms without apparent reason. From her mother's concurrent analysis her therapist learned that Ann's relapse had set in "on the morning after the mother had visited her gynaecologist for a check-up. On the way home from the doctor the mother had the fleeting thought that Ann might have a recurrence of her phobia because she remembered that Ann's original phobia had started almost one and a half years ago on the day after she had visited the same doctor."

An important series of observations reported by S. A. Szurek and A. M. Johnson[127] point in the same direction. Systematic studies of mothers and children in the course of what the authors describe as collaborative psychotherapy showed that the parent's repressed impulses may be acted out by their offspring in a striking way. They may thus be responsible for such behaviour difficulties as truancy, stealing or sexual aberrations. But the authors do not indicate the way in which the child becomes aware of such repressed and unconscious impulses in his parent.

Dr. Sperling specifically rejects the telepathy hypothesis to account for such observations. She tries to show that the unconscious wishes of the mother transmitted themselves to the child through some "concrete signs which could be received by the child through ordinary sensory perception." H. Deutsch[26] in her study of the Psychology of Women has expressed a similar view. So has D. Burlingham[17] in a paper devoted to the empathic response of infants in relation to their mothers. But it is difficult to apply such an explanation to the early infantile period when neural pathways are as yet incompletely developed. There is general consensus that the infant, in the first few months of his life, does not possess an ego of his own—that is to say, his motor and sensory functions show only a very poor degree of organization. This is also one of the conclusions drawn from Dr. Spitz's observations. He states specifically that in the infant "the defence functions of the ego are replaced by a high perceptive threshold and a quasi-biological unity with his mother." If this is true it is difficult to understand how the available data can be reconciled with the assumption that the infant should possess at the same time such unusual powers of observation as some psychologists are inclined to attribute to him.

Again, even if we are prepared to accept the hypothesis of the child's hypersensitiveness to minute sensory clues given to him by the significant adult this does not explain the striking impact of such influences upon his behaviour. Indeed, most observations quoted in the literature indicate that his responses to clues of this kind are far in excess of his usual reactions to overt behaviour encountered in his social environment.

It is at this point that the telepathy hypothesis can fill the gap in our understanding. Once the experimental findings discussed in the preceding chapter are taken for granted, observations like those reported by Rene Spitz, Melitta Sperling or Flanders Dunbar are readily understood. We may assume that in Dunbar's case the child's visual or auditory response to her aunt's attitude was supplemented by a telepathic factor. The same considerations apply to Barbara's reaction to her mother's unconscious hostile wishes directed against her. It is true that in the absence of tracer effects in all these cases the telepathic nature of the incidents described is impossible to prove. But so is the hypothesis of the child's responses to infinitesimal sensory clues; of emotional contagion, empathy or what not. In fact, I hinted that in the case of the young infant the hypothesis of his hypersensitiveness to highly structured sensory impressions is inapplicable.

If this is understood we may just as well take one more

guarded step in the way of analogous reasoning. Why should the infant's unconscious responses to the significant adult be confined to such pathological reactions as were discussed so far? We have rather to assume that virtually all formative stimuli originating from the child's social environment follow the same pattern. They are transmitted to him on two or three functional levels simultaneously, with telepathy playing the most significant part at the pre-verbal level of communication. Indeed, we may assume that at this stage telepathy serves a compelling biological need and represents a functional link between mother and child *here* and *now*, comparable to the function of instinct which, according to current concepts, forms the connecting link between successive generations in the longitudinal section of our racial history.

T. Benedek[9], in a recent article dealing with the psycho-somatic implications of the "primary unit: mother and child," arrives at similar conclusions. She considers the mother-child relationship as a direct continuation of the symbiosis which exists between the two during pregnancy. At this early stage it would indeed be futile to argue to what extent they may be regarded as two separate biological entities. Again, even at a later stage the separation of the infant from the maternal organism is only a matter of degree. It could be stated that so far as his metabolism is concerned the baby nursing on his mother's breast has made but one faltering step beyond the phase when his meals were provided through the passage of placental blood to his circulation in pre-natal life.

There is in this way but a slow and gradual transition from feeding on substances drawn directly from the maternal organism to feeding on substances derived from the outer world. In a similar vein the gradual development of the child's ego is contingent upon his capacity to take in and digest *mental content* originating from sources other than parental figures and transmitted to him on the *psi* level. Prior to this stage we must assume that there is a well-nigh unlimited two-way flow of mental content passing between parent and child without the need for such intermediary steps of catapsychic disorganization of the material as to which I referred in Chapter X.

Yet as time goes on, with the gradual maturation of his ego functions, the child becomes increasingly impervious to heteropsychic influences. His relationship to his mother ceases to be exclusively guided and controlled by *psi* factors, by enkinetic and empathic responses to subliminal sensory stimuli. More and more it assumes the character of conscious communication. It is at this point that he may voice his protest against too rigid a regime of toilet training; against an overpunctilious feeding schedule. He may insist on moving his bowels or emptying his bladder at his own discretion; on having his pudding or his milkshake at his leisure and on his own terms. He may resist his mother's unconscious drive for continued dominance and set his claim for a detached, self-contained autonomous existence against her continued need for an expanded ego. He may fly into tempers when thwarted; he may be naughty; he may seek to be himself: a human being in his own right.

But this is also the time when, as a result of his isolation from his mother—and thereby from nature at large—he may first experience pangs of anxiety and the sense of loneliness as an individual human being. By now he should, however, have also acquired the means of emerging from his isolation. He should be able to establish a new kind of contact with his social environment: his relationship with his fellows shifts to his operating on the ego level. It is true that from now on these same ego functions stand in the way of his previous ability to communicate with his elders on the *psi* level. We have reason to assume that whatever impressions emanating from them do continue to pass through the protective barriers of his personality structure are subjected to the process of catapsychic breakdown and disorganization before they are capable of being assimilated by his ego. He may still "sense" his parents' approval or disapproval in an empathic way. He may still be the recipient of formative stimuli promoting growth and encouraging action, or of "messages" amounting to restrictive taboos and injunctions on a non-verbal level. But he has already learned to focus attention on language and meaning and developed the skill to communicate with those around him with the help of symbols. In this way, while the animal ties by which he had been linked to the maternal organism are subject to gradual obliteration, he enters into a new functional relationship with society—into one based on the give-and-take of intelligent communication, of controlled responses to the intricate system of clues upon which our culture is based. He becomes part of a family group, of a community of playmates, friends, and neighbours. The days of his isolation from the world around him are over. He is a social being operating on the ego level, while the major portion of his potentialities of functioning on the *psi* level recedes into the background.

In summary, it can be stated that on a deeper level the child-parent relationship is based on empathic responses and on the tendency to vicarious functioning operating between the two. These attitudes may manifest themselves in patterns of sharing involving such vital processes as emotional growth, learning, and accommodation to social demands and cultural mores current in the child's environment. They may be instrumental in what has been called the development of the social character. Or else they may result in patterns of resistance, indicative of the child's struggle to sever the bonds still tying him to his mother's personality and to become a self-contained and detached individual in his own right. In the last analysis, patterns of sharing tend toward perpetuation of family traits. They are the psychological equivalents of hereditary transmission. Conversely, it is the pattern of resisting which is ultimately responsible for change in cultural patterns. It is the psychological counterpart of mutations studied by the geneticist.

In both cases there is reason to believe that a telepathic factor is involved in the child-parent relationship even though its operation is rarely amenable to proof by statistical methods.

CHAPTER XIV

Patterns of Neurotic Interaction

THE study of the child-mother relationship rightly occupies the prime place in modern dynamic psychiatry, social psychology and anthropology. It stands as a model of interpersonal relationships in general from which all subsequent patterns of social interaction and interdependence can be derived. The inescapable conflict created by the need to break up the original biological unity between mother and child is thus a basic feature of the human situation, transcending the limitations of any particular culture or historical period.

The stage for the conflict is set as soon as the child's growth into a self-contained and self-directed personality in its own right meets with its parent's instinctive need to maintain her hold over her offspring. In the extreme case the child's determined effort to break away from the fetters of a possessive mother constitutes an irresistible force. But her desire for continued control over what she still considers part and parcel of her own body image may become an immovable object which can ultimately break his will and leave him with a stunted capacity for growth.

But I have emphasized that there also is a positive side to the picture. Patterns of conflict and resistance go hand in hand with patterns of empathic and enkinetic sharing which, I indicated, are responsible for the continuity of tradition and the persistence of mores in our culture.

Viewed from our angle, patterns of sharing and resistance can be traced throughout the three principal levels of personality structure: throughout the ego, the id, and the *psi* level. This is particularly obvious when we turn our attention to the various distortions and exaggerations of these patterns that can be seen in neurotic family situations. But we shall also see that such patterns are often combined with complementary reactions of various types and shades, including attitudes of submission versus dominance, or competitive self-assertion versus passivity and surrender. It may also be recalled that, focusing on the *psi* level, the relationship between the paranoic patient and his alleged persecutor can also be described in terms of complementary reactions. Such psychotic distortions of interaction were discussed in a previous study[32] and can be disregarded in the present context.

The case histories that follow are chosen to illustrate the three principal neurotic patterns to which we have just referred.

Mrs. L., an obsessive compulsive mother aged thirty-six, has difficulties with her son's toilet training. At the age of two Merril still refuses to have his bowel movements on the potty and screams whenever forced to do so. He soils himself promptly when put into his crib or playpen. He sucks his thumb so persistently that his mother consulted a dentist about possible damage to the child's teeth. The dentist advised her to take Merril to a child psychiatrist who in turn recommended psychotherapy for Mrs. L.

It soon became apparent that Merril's eliminative functions had become a source of annoyance and repulsion to his mother's perfectionist trend. She had herself been an only child, brought up by a doting father and a cold and egotistic mother. Her only playmate was a cousin of about her own age and she recalls her violent jealousy of what she felt was his privileged position as a boy. She despised her mother who, in her eyes, was "just" a woman, and formed a strong fixation on her father whom she admired and whom she tried to emulate in many ways. It was obvious that she regarded her son more as a rival than as a child of her own and that she was jealous of the attention her husband paid to him.

Here, too, as in the cases described in the previous chapter, the child responded to his mother's attitude as though he had known as much about her conflicts as a trained psychiatrist. In the first and second years of life his defiance manifested itself on the anal and oral levels. In the second and third year he developed another symptom. Although otherwise of normal intelligence Merril was backward at speaking and had only a few articulated words at his command. His mother's frantic attempts to make him speak were of no avail. He was mute in her company. Yet it was noted that "when left alone" he was able to use words which he never uttered in his mother's presence.

The neurotic nature of Merril's retardation became obvious when his condition improved as soon as Mrs. L. was given psychological treatment. After three months she had gained a modicum of control over her compulsive drives. At the same time Merril became completely toilet trained and gave up his excessive thumb-sucking. His progress remained slow on the verbal level.

It is interesting to note that the apparent improvement of his mother's neurosis was accompanied by a temporary exacerbation of a duodenal ulcer from which she had been suffering. On becoming aware of her hostility towards her son she had forced on herself a greater degree of self-control than she could cope with at that stage and this accounted for the shift of symptoms from the prevailing obsessive compulsive to the psychosomatic side.

It goes without saying that the part played by telepathy versus empathy, enkinesis, etc., must remain a matter for speculation in highly complex clinical constellations of this order. Observations like these can be accounted for by reference to the familiar standby of subliminal sensory clues, emotional contagion, or the like. But even though it cannot be corroborated by reference to clear-cut tracer effects, telepathy as an added means of unconscious communication may well serve as a legitimate auxiliary hypothesis for a better understanding of the dynamics involved.

The following more detailed case history throws light on the neurotic struggle between mother, son, and daughter, observed at a later stage. Sylvia is a woman of forty-five, suffering from an obsessive compulsive neurosis. Of Irish Catholic descent, she was brought up in an atmosphere of repression and Victorian respectability. An only brother, two years her junior, was the favourite of the family. He surpassed her both at childish games at home, on the playground, and at school. While it was understood that he was to go to college and was destined for a brilliant career she was to stay at home and to prepare for married life. Although of pleasant appearance, Sylvia was shy and self-conscious with boys, had few dates and ultimately accepted a suitor selected by her parents. Her marriage soon proved a failure. Sylvia was fearful and frigid during intercourse and found to her dismay that her husband was suffering from premature ejaculation. She came to despise him for his inability to satisfy her sexually, and suspected him of having married her solely for monetary reasons. The birth of two children in an interval of two years failed to close the rift between them. She was strict and controlling with Donald, the younger child, and permissive and indulgent with Rosalyn, two years Don's senior.

On reaching high-school age Don was sent to an expensive boarding school while Rosalyn stayed with her mother. Following Don's departure Sylvia became increasingly concerned with his health. She developed a variety of obsessive compulsive symptoms which were aggravated whenever he returned from boarding school. She anxiously watched his eating habits and was thrown into panic when she noticed that his appetite was below par, or when he seemed pale or listless. Such observations would start a chain of fearful ruminations ending with the conclusion that he was gravely ill and going to die from stomach-bleeding like his father. She would question herself whether she had prepared his meals the right way, whether the meat was tender enough, whether fats used were easily digestible and any canned food served really safe for consumption.

Don proved to be a gifted child but showed little interest in his studies. He remained impassive to his mother's constant prodding, sought to avoid competitive games, and drove her to desperation with his indifference and lack of ambition. She wanted him to become both an athlete and a successful scholar and was disappointed with what she called his sissyish behaviour. All these traits, she confessed later, reminded her of her weak and inefficient husband. She became increasingly impatient with the boy and sought to force on him a more vigorous and more masculine regime. At the same time she harassed her family doctor with detailed accounts of various imaginary symptoms of disease which she thought she observed in the boy. She became panicky when he failed to write to her every day and would telephone the school in the middle of the night to find out how he was.

Rosalyn, by contrast, became a meek, submissive child. She complied in every way with her mother's wishes. In her later teens it became evident that she had adopted much of Sylvia's compulsive pattern. She imitated her neurotic mannerisms, showed the identical ambivalence conflicts when faced with decisions, duplicated all her perfectionistic trends, and suffered from the same feeling of harassment in relation to the lapse of time. Mother and daughter would consult each other about their shopping and go through the same interminable obsessive ruminations in relation to every item. Though different in their physical appearance, the resemblance in their general demeanour was unmistakable.

Analysis soon revealed the deeper roots of Sylvia's anxiety concerning Don. She had numerous sadistic-aggressive fantasies in connection with him, some of them with a castrating content. It was obvious that she was identifying him both with her deceased husband and with her brother, who had outshone her in childhood years because he was stronger, smarter and more popular than she and, above all, because he was a boy. Her unhappy marital relationship was a second traumatic experience, superimposed on painful memories of early sibling rivalry. It was aggravated by her husband's failure to make up for what she felt was her basic shortcoming by compensating her with his own masculine prowess. Growing up without male prerogatives—without a penis, as it were—was bad enough. Having her hopes dashed of being supplied with a second-hand penis was an additional frustration which touched off the first adult manifestation of her neurosis. Her son's shortcomings, true or imaginary, threw salt on the old wound and reactivated her infantile conflict.

Some of Sylvia's fantasies were of a masochistic nature. She saw herself as a slave tortured by brutal males. Her hands and feet were tied and she was utterly helpless. Sometimes she replaced male tormentors by women.

In her sadistic fantasies she took revenge on the rival of her childhood years. She took possession of, or disposed of the symbol of his hateful masculine superiority. Her dreams reflected the same aggressive attitude towards her son and her husband. They showed her on the search for a lost motor-car, for keys she had mislaid, for a handbag that had been stolen. Some dreams contained references to homosexual fantasies in which she assumed the role of the masculine partner.

Her cruel fantasies provoked inevitable feelings of guilt which in turn accounted for her exaggerated solicitude for Don's welfare. Yet she had also another reason to see him strong, masculine, and aggressive: he was destined to be a living antidote to her own feeling of feminine inferiority. Fate which had deprived her of a penis—or at least of a sexually potent husband—had given her another chance and she was determined to make the best of it this time. In this way Don had not only become a reincarnation of both a rival and a frustrating figure from the past. He also was her best hope for the future, the only one holding the promise of realizing, at long last, her dream of masculine superiority, by proxy, as it were.

This explains her ambitious plans for Don's education. On finishing his high school she placed him in one of the leading colleges of the country, hoping he would develop his undeniable talent for an academic career. A devout Catholic, she took it also for granted that he would follow in her footsteps and embrace the same religious outlook and philosophy. All the deeper was her disappointment when she realized his utter indifference towards her ambitious schemes. He was at best a mediocre student, poor at games and physical training, and offered continued passive resistance to her prodding.

Don's personality thus seemed to develop into the diametrical opposite of his mother's. Although greatly concerned with matters pertaining to his physical comfort he was never in a hurry, never rushed. Never a diligent churchgoer, he showed sympathies with "leftish" views and chose his friends among politically radical elements of the college. At twenty-two he surprised Sylvia with the news that he had become engaged to marry a Jewish college girl, a year older than himself.

His mother responded with renewed exacerbation of her neurosis, aggravated by gastro-intestinal symptoms. In one of her dreams dreamt at that time she saw herself at her son's wedding. The flowers were brought in on a hearse, which gave her the feeling of impending doom—perhaps of Don's death. But on the following night she dreamt she had given his bride a wedding gown designed by herself. She was anxious the gown should fit the bride and that the bride should be happy wearing it. In another dream she saw herself and her son's fiancée in mortal danger. She felt she could avert the danger if she could only remember a certain sentence which she would have to say.

On the night of the wedding she had an attack of gastro-enteritis. It reappeared on the return of the newly-weds from their honeymoon. It was apparent that she had been watching for whatever clues to Don's marital life she could glean with the same anxiety as she had shown in relation to his digestive and eliminative functions and his physical welfare in general.

This condensed account of Sylvia's case may suffice in the present connection. It is chosen to illustrate her compulsive need to make up for what she felt were her son's shortcomings with an excessive tendency to enkinesis or vicarious functioning. This tendency manifested itself in her neurotic concern, first, over his eliminative functions; secondly, over his eating habits, thirdly, over his sex life. Prompted by her own past deprivations, especially in the sexual sphere, her whole life was devoted to one purpose: to make up for her frustrations. To her unconscious Don remained nothing but a detached part of her own personality. Thus it was quite consistent when she sought to use him as a tool for the realization of her own life goals. Whether we describe this attitude as identification or a tendency to vicarious functioning or enkinesis is immaterial. The fact is that to her Don never ceased to be a direct extension of her personality, an appendage to her body image. She had never relinquished the claim for exclusive control of his bodily functions—alimentary, urogenital or otherwise—as though they were her own. Whenever she found him failing in his responses to a given situation she would react with the same frustration and anger which can occasionally be seen in a hemiplegic seeking to move a paralysed limb.

Is there any evidence that Sylvia's tendency to vicarious

functioning has in actual fact made an impact upon her son's behaviour which cannot be accounted for by reference to the "usual channels of sensation"? Are there any tracer effects in Don's case history upon which such an argument can be based? Don was seen by the present writer in a few interviews only which threw but little light on the psychodynamics involved on his side. But there is one significant fact that emerged: Don's sex life had been rather inhibited up to the time of his marriage. Haunted by castration fear he refrained from masturbation until the age of fourteen or fifteen, when it was accompanied by masochistic phantasies. In others he would imagine himself to subject his partner—a slave girl—to various cruel practices. The reader will recall that fantasies of the same kind played a prominent part in his mother's neurosis.

Otherwise Don showed no overt symptoms of neurosis and achieved satisfactory adjustment both to his married and professional life.

Whatever levels of interaction were involved in Sylvia's relationship to her children, it is thus obvious that they responded to her in two contrasting ways. While Rosalyn's neurosis can be described in terms of empathic and enkinetic sharing of her mother's obsessive compulsive trend, Don's reaction is an example of resistance to Sylvia's exaggerated enkinetic attitudes. The ultimate reason for this early cleavage must remain a matter of conjecture. Its importance for the ultimate character formation of Sylvia's offspring cannot, however, be over-estimated. It may well be that it was Rosalyn's tendency to sharing and submitting to her mother's compulsive standards which paved the way for her own neurotic personality deviation, while Don's resistance to and rebellion against the same parental attitude saved him from more serious damage to his personality.

The following observation throws more light upon the dynamics underlying patterns of neurotic sharing. Mrs. S. was suffering from frigidity as part of her obsessive compulsive trend. One of her symptoms was excessive concern over cleanliness and sphincter control. She had marked anal guilt, connected with early difficulties in her toilet training. An isolated incident of bedwetting at the age of fifteen was particularly humiliating to her. Subsequently, she was afraid that she might lose urine during intercourse. To her painful embarrassment this had actually occurred during her wedding night. Since that time her fear of wetting had grown to phobic proportions severely affecting her sexual adjustment.

Mrs. S.'s problem was not, however, the only neurotic difficulty in her family. Victor, her only son, a bright and well-developed child of eight, was suffering from persistent bed-wetting. Yet despite her apparent anger over his enuresis, and in contrast to her intolerance with occasional other misdemeanours, Mrs. S. was unusually permissive in regard to Victor's wetting habit and failed to do anything about it until the beginning of her own treatment. The reason for this was brought out by her analysis. It showed that the patient's compulsive cleanliness was a typical reaction formation to her own problems concerned with eliminatory functions. Her permissiveness in relation to her son's enuresis was in part determined by her own repressed instinctual needs and thus helped to perpetuate the pattern of neurotic sharing between the two. Victor was seen by the present writer in two diagnostic interviews. They revealed the child's obstinate resistance to his mother's compulsive trend, although his rebellion was masked by his outwardly compliant behaviour. It was decided that psychotherapy with the boy should be deferred until more progress was achieved with his mother. Three months later Mrs. S. had the following dream: "I am in my childhood home. I see a faucet and want to turn off the water. I turn it one way, then the other way but I can't turn it off. I get frantic and give it a big turn. But now the water just pours more than before and splashes all over the place. Mother and father are there. Mother is quite upset; she says 'My Goodness, look what you have done.' But I see only a few drops on the floor and tell her so. 'Look, only a few drops, so why are you so upset?' "

The dream occurred following intercourse with her husband and shows the patient's confusion about genital and urinary functions. At the same time her attempt to turn off the faucet indicates that she is trying hard to relinquish her infantile, pregenital, method of sexual gratification to which she had clung in the past in defiance of both her mother and her husband. On a more superficial level the dream expresses her identification with her son and with his problem of bedwetting.

In this case it appears that psychotherapy had succeeded in making a dent in the existing pattern of sharing. Mrs. S. was given an interpretation of the dream and she left my office visibly moved, feeling that an important milestone had been reached in her analysis. In the next session, a week after the dream described, she surprised me with the report that Victor, for the first time since she could remember, had been dry during the whole week. Apart from two or three minor accidents his improvement has been maintained during the past six months. Whether and how far telepathy was involved in this development must, in the absence of unequivocal tracer elements, remain a matter for speculation.

CHAPTER XV

Complementary Neuroses

With a Note on Psi Factors in Mating and Marriage

THE types of neurotic interaction described in the previous chapter were discussed with special reference to patterns of sharing and resisting in a given family situation. But Sylvia's relationship to her son, Donald, or that of Mrs. S. to Victor, is at the same time a good illustration of the complementary type of neurotic interaction. Such patterns were described by B. Mittelmann[83] in persons living in intimate relationships, especially in marriage partners. They are also suggested by the observations of C. P. Oberndorf,[90] E. Bergler,[10] S. A. Szurek and A. M. Johnson,[127] M. Sperling,[120] and many others.

Complementary neurotic patterns, in some cases, give the impression of an intrapsychic conflict projected back into the outside world. They may amount to a re-enaction by new protagonists of the early infantile conflicts from which, according to current psychoanalytical concepts, they were originally derived. The contrasting characterological pictures created in such family situations may be unmistakable even to the psychologically untrained observer. The neurosis of one member of the family group may appear to fit the neurosis of another member like tongue and groove, like the hand fits the glove, or, to quote a phrase used by Franz Kafka, like the arrow fits the wound.

The following case history illustrates the father's role in a neurotic family situation, reminiscent, in a small way, of Kafka's own distorted relationship to his father. Edgar N., aged twenty, was the only son of a successful lawyer and of a doting over-solicitous mother. Mr. N., a self-made man, worked his way up the social scale at the price of occasional attacks of duodenal ulcer. Despite his show of self-assurance and of a forceful personality he was subject to depressions and anxiety states. Edgar grew up in a poor proletarian district of a large mid-western city, amid tough "dead-end kids" who gave him a rough time when joining their games in the streets and backyards of the neighbourhood. Although closely resembling his well-built athletic father he was of frail physique, shy and inhibited with strangers. His movements were clumsy, he was poor at sports and never stood up to a fight with boys of his age. Rejected by the group he withdrew into his shell, became a voracious reader, intellectually precocious, a model child. Yet at the age of ten he was still dependent on his mother for dressing, washing, and bathing and it was at the public toilet at high school that he first noticed that other boys did not clean themselves following defaecation in an upright position—a habit he had maintained from the time of his toilet training.

His father, realizing Edgar's excessive dependent needs, tried his best to help him to become the active, out-going, aggressive boy Mr. N. himself had been in his youth. He was deeply concerned over Edgar's shortcomings. He felt them as a blow to his own self-esteem and considered Edgar's failure in life as a failure of his own. Mr. N. joined the boys of the street gang at their ball games, showed them his ways of batting and pitching, of wrestling and boxing. Yet Edgar, instead of benefiting from his father's well-intended efforts, became increasingly timid and withdrawn. He gave up hope of ever keeping pace with boys of his age, to say nothing of competing with a man like his father on a mature level. He sought refuge in the world of books and later in day-dreams and fantasies. He saw himself as a great writer, scientist or philosopher. On his father's insistance he reluctantly joined the Boy Scouts but failed at simple tests he was expected to pass. His father retaliated with a ban on reading. Edgar, in turn, broke the ban by taking his books at night under his blanket, reading with the aid of a flashlight.

At the age of eleven he wrote an impassioned letter, accusing his father of robbing him of his freedom of "thought and action" and insisting on his "right" to keep away from the Boy

Scouts, to withdraw from the group and to hold on to his neurotic pattern of defence in general. In analysis Edgar reported the following recurrent dream: "I am walking with my father on a plain. There are many cracks in the ground. Suddenly father's foot is caught in one of the cracks; the crack gives in, he is caught between the edges. He falls into the chasm." In one of his early recollections Edgar's father chases him around the table to punish him for a minor misdemeanour. Suddenly Edgar turns against him shouting, "You big bully, you," whereupon father gives up the chase. His fantasies were of a bizarre sado-masochistic nature but he refrained from overt masturbatory activities. The Oedipal conflict dominated the picture, combined with thinly veiled incestuous fantasies relating to his mother. This accounts for his profound castration fears as illustrated by the following dream: "There is an ugly piece of flesh coming out of my face. It has the shape of a penis jutting out of my right cheek." Edgar's associations in connection with this dream led him back to a scene in his childhood when a dog jumped at him and bit his right cheek. He yelled, "Mummy, I will die, I will die." He recalled his mother's fears that he would be disfigured for life.

Edgar's sex life was rudimentary. At about nineteen he had made an abortive attempt at intercourse with a girl with whom he had not been emotionally involved. Following a necking party with another girl he dreamt that while kissing her his tongue disintegrated in his mouth. Here, again, the presence of castration anxiety is unmistakable.

Safely entrenched in a position of withdrawal from both work and social responsibilities Edgar entered the therapeutic relationship as what he called an "interested onlooker." He came to oblige his father but made it clear that he saw no need to change his ways; he felt quite happy and secure in the impasse which he had reached. He explained that defying his father and counteracting every move which he planned for his son was a matter of self-respect for him. He admitted that so long as his wish to choose an academic career met with Mr. N.'s resistance he had been keenly interested in literary and philosophical matters. But as soon as his father had become agreeable to Edgar's wishes he stalled, lost interest and, like a motor-car in the absence of friction, actually came to a standstill. The same thing happened when his father started prodding him "to pick up a girl and to have a good time with her." This only gave Edgar the feeling that sex was another task at which he had no chance to compete with his father and reinforced his pattern of withdrawal.

There were few areas in Edgar's life which were not vitiated by his unfortunate relationship with his parents. Accordingly one of the first objectives of the treatment was the establishment of a new relationship, free from parental pressures, in which the futility of his fears and guilt feelings could be brought home to the patient. It is significant that here, too, it was difficult to protect Edgar from his father's excessive anxiety to "help"—that is, to function vicariously on his behalf. Even though he realized that he should temporarily step out of the picture, Mr. N. sought to enlist the analyst to take over his role. Telephone calls giving specific advice concerning what Edgar was or was not supposed to do and in what way the analyst should seek to bring his weight to bear on the patient were the order of the day. It was obvious that Mr. N. was himself suffering from a compulsion neurosis comparable to the one described in Sylvia, the mother of Don and Rosalyn.

Edgar responded well to analytic treatment. He was soon able to express his hostility against his father and gradually lost his fears in competitive life situations. By the end of one year's treatment a major part of his conflicts was resolved and his castration anxiety dissipated.

His father seemed to be overjoyed by Edgar's progress. Yet it was at this time, at about the ninth month of the treatment, that Mr. N. developed increasing symptoms of gastric distress. It was diagnosed as due to a recently developed duodenal ulcer. There could be little doubt that he was unable to accept Edgar's newly won independence from parental control. As in the case of Merril's mother, described in the preceding chapter, Mr. N.'s occasional contacts with the therapist had made him aware of his unconscious hostility towards his son and his frantic effort to keep these impulses under control precipitated the development of his somatic symptoms. Yet he remained unwilling to face the ambivalent nature of his feelings for his only child. He was sure that nothing but Edgar's welfare had been uppermost in his mind.

It is interesting to note that Edgar himself responded with guilt feelings to his father's gastric symptoms. He confessed that on repeated occasions he had the fantasy of hitting Mr. N.'s abdomen with his fist and he asked himself whether this had not been a factor contributing to the development of his ulcers. The therapist hastened to reassure Edgar on this score—although he has to admit that he did so with an element of doubt which perhaps is understandable in the light of the subject-matter discussed here.

* * *

Neurotic family situations involving several members of the family are illustrated by the following brief observations. Catherine was an unmarried woman of twenty-five. As an only child she had become the confidante of her mother at a tender age. Frustrated in her marriage to a weak and sexually inadequate husband, her mother revealed intimate details of her married life to her daughter. Catherine grew up to become keenly interested in boyish games, scornful of the feminine ways of her schoolmates, and developed marked athletic prowess, together with thinly veiled homosexual tendencies that made her seek the role of masculine superiority in her affairs with men. It was evident that she had chosen to play the very role in life at which her father had failed her mother. She became a "career" woman and a latent homosexual. Yet there is no doubt that describing Catherine's attitude in terms of masculine protest, penis envy, or the like, gives only partly justice to her case. Such a description would pay no attention to the dynamics of her complementary reaction to her father's shortcomings which played such an important part in the development of her character structure.

The part played by sibling rivalry in the development of neurotic patterns has already been brought out in the dynamics of Sylvia's obsessive compulsive neurosis. It is further illustrated by the following case. Eleanor was a woman of thirty-one whose chief problem consisted of an overt homosexual trend. She grew up in constant competition with a brother, four years her junior. At the age of four, little Tony had an accident and sustained injury to his tongue. He was left with a bad speech defect throughout his childhood and adolescent years. Eleanor, in turn, developed into a fluent talker, stealing the show from both boys and girls wherever she went; she won prizes in elocution and made the stage her career. Her lifelong competition with an insignificant sibling was indeed crowned by success. But for this she had to pay with a profound deviation of her psychosexual development.

That the clash of wills between parent and child may occasionally extend to the deepest levels of the personality structure and lead to a characteristic complementary pattern of psychosomatic symptoms is shown by the following observation. Tilda was an unmarried woman of thirty, the oldest of six siblings. She grew up in circumstances of squalor and poverty which were chiefly the fault of her weak and sub-intelligent mother who, in addition, was suffering from periodic melancholia. During such spells she would pass into a semi-stuporous condition, develop faulty habits, and lose control of her bladder. Tilda succeeded in breaking away from her family, worked her way through high school and college and became a registered nurse in charge of a children's ward in a big hospital until she had to quit her job owing to repeated conflicts with her superiors. Tilda's difficulties showed a distinctly neurotic pattern for which she sought help through psychotherapy. Her sexual adjustment was seriously disturbed. She was unable to accept her feminine role, was ashamed of the size of her breasts (which were in no way conspicuous) and was hostile and aggressive in her relations to men.

Psychotherapy helped her to gain a more detached attitude towards her family and especially her mother. After an absence of twelve years during which time she had helped them by financial support she decided to pay a visit to her widowed mother and to see for herself what could be done about the desperate family situation. She found the house in a condition worse than expected. It was pervaded by the familiar odour of urine. Her mother was obviously back in one of her spells of melancholia and suffered from incontinence of the bladder. Yet she obstinately refused to be seen by a doctor. The younger children, incapable of coping with the situation, let things go from bad to worse and implored the older sister to make arrangements for the mother's commitment.

Shocked by the plight of her family Tilda tried her best to persuade her mother to seek medical help and to accept hospitalization. But, as in years past, she found herself unable to take a firm stand. On the second day of her stay at home, she was laid up by a sudden illness. She was unable to pass water for nearly twelve hours and developed severe pain in the lower abdominal region. Catheterization revealed a spasm of the sphincters of her urinary bladder and evidence of an acute non-specific cystitis.

Tilda turned for assistance to a district nurse and cut her stay in her home town shorter than contemplated. After a week she returned to New York for treatment of her cystitis. It should be noted at this point that there is no previous history of cystitis in her case nor could the source of her bladder infection be ascertained by careful medical examination. Evidently it was the shock suffered by the sight of her incontinent mother which had mobilized her need to function vicariously in her behalf, causing spasm of the sphincter muscles and urinary retention, followed by infection. Yet it should also be noted that this type of psychosomatic response is not the only one which could be observed in Tilda's case. Such occasional symptoms as muscular rigidities, abdominal cramps, etc., were expressions of intrapsychic conflicts confined more strictly to the autopsychic sphere. Her excessive reaction to her mother's infirmity followed the same pattern extending, however, into the heteropsychic sphere.

Similar reactions are by no means rare, as can be seen in the following case. Dora was a married woman of twenty-four, suffering from severe premenstrual and menstrual cramps, causing her uterus to become a hard tumour-like mass in her abdomen. During menstruation she was invariably constipated for several days. There is also evidence of marked sexual maladjustment connected with a deep-seated confusion regarding the relationship of death and sexual activities and with guilt feelings over loss of sphincter control. Her analysis also revealed that since Dora could remember, her mother had been suffering from severe menstrual bleeding. Following the birth of a younger sister when Dora was seven years old, hysterectomy had to be performed. Dora recalled the days which she spent by her mother's bedside, terrified lest the haemorrhage would recur and she would have to do something about it—she did not exactly know what.

These early experiences, superimposed on infantile conflicts arising from her toilet training by a compulsive mother, made Dora's first menstruation a major shock. She took it for an exact repetition of what she thought had been her mother's incurable malady. From then onward Dora "tightened up" every month; she developed cramps, sought to stop the haemorrhage—and very nearly succeeded in doing so. She developed her pattern of dysmenorrhoea and spastic constipation which were the presenting symptoms of her neurosis in the somatic sphere.

Certainly, this brief account gives only a partial picture of Dora's problems, but it shows that here, again, the choice of the affected organ was largely determined by her mother's illness and by the way the latter had responded to her own genital bleedings. It is significant that an older sister who had been exposed to similar childhood experiences was also suffering from severe menstrual cramps, whereas the younger sister, after whose birth hysterectomy had to be performed in Dora's mother, was spared any menstrual discomfort.

* * *

Reports of telepathic interaction and intercommunication, both spontaneous and experimental, between marriage partners abound in the literature of psychical research,[52, 87] and need not be discussed in the present context. Nor is it necessary to elaborate the countless modern versions of the age-old theme of love "conquering the barriers of time and space" featured in folk-lore and poetic fiction of all times.

But the following case of telepathy between husband and wife may be described here as an example of the enkinetic attitude of one spouse getting "through" to the other on the dream level, as it were. Mr. L., a German scholar living in the United States, was preparing an historical study of Lenin's secret entry into Russia at the end of World War I. His article contained a reference to the famous *Panzerzug* the German General Staff had put at Lenin's disposal. But Mr. L., working from German sources, was at a loss to find the English equivalent for *Panzerzug*. The hour was late. Too tired to consult his dictionary he decided to do so in the morning. Still haunted by the missing word he went to bed and fell asleep. Mrs. L., his wife, had gone to bed a few hours before him. She had been unaware of the paper her husband had been writing and knew nothing of his particular linguistic problem. Nor was her command of the English language superior to that of Mr. L. First thing in the morning she reported the following dream to Mr. L.: "I heard an utterly ridiculous sentence in my dream. Someone said 'The lady is fair and armoured.' Nothing else." Her husband, dumbfounded, picked up the cue offered to him by the manifest content of the dream. *Armoured* was the key-word he had been vainly looking for the night before.

Mr. and Mrs. L.'s case could not be subjected to analytic exploration. But there can be little doubt of Mrs. L.'s ambitious drive in relation to her husband's career. In her dream she seemed to take the initiative once more, indicating at the same time that she, the "fair lady," did possess the armoured strength which, in her estimate, could do with some reinforcement in his case. Whether or not the word "armoured" represents at the same time a distortion of a more pertinent reference to a lady both *fair* and *enamoured* must remain a matter of speculation.

On the other end of the scale we find patterns of interaction, affecting the deepest levels of personality, including susceptibility to psychosomatic disease. This is illustrated by the following observation. Both spouses in an elderly married couple, attending a psychosomatic clinic, were suffering from bronchial asthma. The wife's history of asthmatic attacks went back to her childhood years. They showed typical seasonal fluctuations due to allergic sensitivity which was ascertained by skin tests. Her husband had lost his job as an ice-block vendor five years ago. Put on relief a year or two later he developed the same asthmatic attacks from which his wife had been suffering for twenty years. Skin tests in his case were negative. His analysis showed the presence of excessive dependent needs which could only be satisfied by competing with his wife for attention that is expected to be paid to an invalid in our culture. As in Tilda's case, described on an earlier page, the patient's choice of symptoms was determined by the existing family pattern. Yet instead of seeking to compensate for an existing defect he responded in terms of identification or empathic and enkinetic sharing—he became his spouse's "partner in sickness."

The following observation comes closer to the pattern of the complementary reaction type. Mr. F., seen in the same clinic, was suffering from ulcerative colitis. At times his diarrhoea was so bad as to overtax his sphincter control and to make him partially incontinent. His wife became more and more constipated as his colitis progressed. Repeated haemorrhoidal attacks required two periods of hospitalization. Finally, haemorrhoidectomy was performed in Mrs. F. During this time Mr. F. had an acute haemorrhage from his colon, also requiring surgical intervention.

Certainly, these are extreme examples of two alternative neurotic reaction types as they occur among individuals living together in a closely knit family relationship. But they bring a basic pattern into sharper focus which easily escapes attention in less pronounced cases. Such cases are the object of B. Mittelmann's[83] study of complementary neuroses in marriage partners, mentioned in a previous chapter. Mittelmann calls attention to the fact that reactions of this type may at times afford relief to one of the spouses involved. Alternatively, they may perpetuate the existing pathology by setting up a vicious circle which can only be broken by the treatment of both spouses.

E. Bergler,[10] on the other hand, has pointed out that interlacing patterns of dominance versus submission may be important factors in the choice of marriage partners. The striking fact is that one neurotic suffering from a latent sadistic trend may be attracted to his masochistic counterpart with the unfailing instinct of a homing salmon making his way to his native creek. Every experienced psychiatrist knows of cases in which one sadistic partner may try his luck with one masochistic partner after the other—although no one seems to be able to tell how such a choice can be made without submitting the prospective spouse to a preliminary Szondi test.

The same problem is highlighted by the following observation. A patient of mine, a bachelor aged thirty, had been involved in one love relationship after another, persistently avoiding marriage. He was suffering from an anxiety neurosis occasioned by all-pervading castration fears. Despite his successes with women he entertained grave doubts about his masculinity, about his sexual prowess and the very physical integrity of his sexual organs. A short time before he commenced treatment he fell "definitely and irrevocably" in love with a girl of twenty-four, who, he said, was the answer to all his prayers. They decided to get engaged. Following their engagement the girl confessed to him her secret. As a sequel to an abdominal infection she had undergone a hysterectomy in her childhood. Her ovaries had to be removed together with the womb. Hormonal treatment successfully masked all symptoms of ovarial deficiency, and my patient could have learned by no conceivable means of observation of his fiancée's affliction so closely resembling what he believed to be an incurable deficiency of his own.

The manner in which we may become aware "in a flash" of another person's latent potentialities in situations of ordinary courtship and mating is no less obscure. What is it that is responsible for "love at first sight"? What is it that makes Romeo reach out among all the maidens in Verona for Juliet so that "touching hers, make blessed my rude hand?" What is it that makes Juliet find Romeo's—and only Romeo's—"gracious self . . . the god of my idolatry"—to the exclusion of all other eligible suitors?

The question has puzzled philosophers, scientists and psychologists from Plato[94] to Theodor Reik.[102] Plato's celebrated fable has it that humans, in bygone times, were four-armed and four-legged beings, sliced into two halves by an irate god. Since then it has been fore-ordained for the two respective halves to look for each other in ceaseless search—so as to become unified wholes again. More modern attempts at theorizing call attention to the mutual attraction seen in persons of like kind (K. Pearson[92]) or, conversely, in people of contrasting personality types (Bain,[7] Ernst Kretschmer,[71] and many others). More recently, L. Szondi[126] devoted an ingenious study to what he described as *Fate Analysis.* In this book he tries to show that the mutual attraction of friends, lovers or marriage partners is ultimately due to hidden "ancestral claims" anchored in the genetic structure of the individual concerned, propelling him or her in the direction of an individual of like genetic structure, even though, on the face of it, this "likeness" may not be discernible to the naked eye. He speaks of a genotropic effect exerted by the similarity of latent or recessive genes. In his view this latent genotropic effect is then responsible especially for such attractions as may determine the choice of one's mate or marriage partner. It may play a decisive part in shaping a person's whole destiny.

This is not the place to go into a discussion of facts and figures upon which Szondi's theory is based. But there is one point which stands out from the vast mass of material which he has collected in its support. His postulated genotropic effect cannot but be perceived in an unconscious way and, as far as living persons are concerned, on the *psi* level. To quote Shakespeare again,

> Lovers and madmen have such seething brains,
> Such shaping fantasies, that apprehend
> More than cool reason ever comprehends.

Certainly, responses to sensory clues also play a part in this process. This is particularly true when Szondi confronts his subjects in artificial test situations with sets of photographs of men and women, asking them to make their selections in their order of preference. But the vast majority of observations upon which Szondi's *Fate Analysis* is based is frankly unintelligible in terms of the classical ego and id psychology—that is, without resort to "shaping fantasies" rooted in deeper levels of the personality structure. Here, too, *psi* may be the connecting link binding the divided parts of Plato's mystical primordial beings together. Or to put it in a somewhat more up-to-date terminology: here, too, telepathy may be the vehicle by which Szondi's hypothetical genotropic effect is brought to bear from person to person and which is ultimately responsible for their mutual attraction, repulsion—or complementary marital neurosis, as the case may be.

CHAPTER XVI

Castration Fear, Superego, and Primal Conflict

A Three-Level Approach

WE have seen that by extending our frame of reference to the *psi* level of interpersonal relationships new light can be thrown on certain aspects of the theory of neuroses and on the dynamics of interpersonal relationships in general. It is in this way that our inquiry leads from the individual to the group, from his personality to his culture. In doing so we have to realize here, again, that we are treading on ground broken many years ago by Freud[44f] and more recently by the culturally oriented schools of psychoanalysis such as those represented by G. Róheim,[106] H. S. Sullivan,[125] Erich Fromm,[46] A. Kardiner,[68] and others. Psychoanalysis, in its original approach, focused attention on the question of socially undesirable, pregenital—anal and oral—drives persisting after the infantile period. It developed the concept of the Oedipus complex and described the gradual emergence of conscience or the superego as the result of the incorporation of parental figures and their moral demands from the outside world into the personality structure. The elaborate picture drawn of the ways in which these repressive and moulding influences are brought to bear upon the child and the adolescent in the course of his upbringing need not be retraced in the present connection.

But there is an important feature in this theory which calls for comment. The original psychoanalytic concept makes ample use of such metaphorical expressions as projection, introjection, identification and the like. It takes the tendency to empathic response, imitative behaviour or emotional contagion for granted and we have seen that it does so even in cases in which it is difficult to tell in what way the host of subtle and often subliminal sensory clues responsible for such reactions can be transmitted from one person to the other. Often reference is made to direct communication between the unconscious of parent and child, implying that the unconscious itself is equipped with a mysterious perceptual apparatus of its own. This, then, was to account for such striking instances of "intuitive" awareness of thoughts, emotions or other mental attitudes that can be observed in many areas of interpersonal relationships, particularly between mother and child, but also between therapist and patient in the psychoanalytic situation.

We already voiced our doubts that such an explanation does justice to the facts. We learn on the one hand of the well-nigh irresistible force of instinctual drives emanating from the id. Yet we should be satisfied, on the other hand, that these drives can be controlled and made to comply with cultural demands by a modulation of voice, by the raising of an eyebrow—if not by the drop of a hat. We observe the appearance of polymorphous sexual drives, of masturbatory activities in early childhood, followed by their gradual obliteration in the ensuing latency period. But in most cases that come to our notice we seek in vain for overt pressures of equal or comparable intensity that could conceivably lead to such results. What we can see are subtle, insiduous influences operating largely on the non-verbal level whose inhibiting effect upon socially undesirable behaviour may be in inverse proportion to the vehemence with which the original drives are looking for outlets.

It is true that we may learn from one or another of our patients that he was literally threatened with castration when caught masturbating as a child. He may recall how his hands were tied to the bedpost to prevent genital play or that he himself believed in the frightful consequences of violating sexual taboos. However, we may also recall the case of Edgar N. discussed in the previous chapter. In this boy any information regarding overt threats to account for his intense castration anxiety was impossible to elicit. His father, when questioned on this point, was perfectly honest in denying that he himself, his wife or anybody else had ever cautioned or intimidated his son. Edgar's own recollection seemed to confirm his father's story. He could not even after prolonged analysis remember anything amounting to overt castration threats. Yet as far as could be ascertained, he had not until his later adolescence indulged in masturbation or engaged in any other overt sexual activity. This in itself may well be taken as a sign of intense castration fears. This is also borne out by the dream quoted on page 175 featuring an early childhood recollection of being bitten by a dog—an experience which Edgar unconsciously connected with the threat of genital mutilation. Observations like these are none too infrequent. Every analyst recalls cases in which to the best of the patient's knowledge castration threats have never been verbalized by his parents or other persons concerned with his upbringing.

Where, then, does the castration fear seen in such persons come from? Fenichel,[37] summarizing older and more recent views on the origin of the castration complex, points out that "in the last analysis the idea of castration may be based upon traces of the ancient biological reflex of autotomy; less deeply but most certainly it is based on the archaic retaliatory idea of talion: the very organ that has sinned has to be punished." Superimposed on these, at bottom hereditary, archetypal factors are in his view the diverse influences emanating from the child's social environment discouraging any and every sexual activity in the pre-adolescent stage.

However, this explanation tacitly implies two presuppositions which are themselves in need of further clarification. First, it presupposes the possibility of hereditary transmission of certain culturally acquired ideas or mental characteristics. This is far from being generally accepted by contemporary psychology. Indeed, H. Hartman and E. Kris,[53] in a recent article, specifically reject Freud's concept of a phylogenetic source of castration fears. Secondly, it implies the possibility that here, again, in the absence of overt castration threats, the child may "sense" in some mysterious way the unformulated and often unconscious hostile tendencies that lie dormant in the minds of his elders.

The observations described in the preceding chapters contain a clue as to the way in which we may assume that such fears are conveyed from parent to offspring: by way of the child's telepathic susceptibility to repressed or preconscious mental content. We have reason to assume that repressed castration tendencies and similar punitive attitudes have become an integral part of the emotional climate which exists in many sectors of our culture. It is precisely because of the unconscious or preconscious nature of these tendencies that they are apt to assume telepathic activity upon the impressionable mind of the child and to exert influences more profound than anything communicated on the verbal level.

However, unconscious hostility harboured by the guardians of "law and order" is not necessarily the only source of anxiety connected with the violation of existing cultural taboos. The same effect may conceivably be brought about by the parents' own repressed fears and communicated to their children on the *psi* level. It is this process which is often described in terms of emotional contagion, leaving the question of the way in which it is transmitted from person to person and, for that matter, from one generation to the other, unanswered.

The same considerations apply to the manner in which influences emanating from parental figures and other persons in authority are responsible for the development of the superego. Psychoanalytic theory holds that parental images are "incorporated" into the child's personality by a process of introjection, whatever this term may mean to indicate. Yet here, too, it is clear that introjection is either merely a figure of speech or tacitly implies telepathy between parent and child, operating on an early developmental level.

If we accept this hypothesis it is readily understood that the superego is usually found to bear the imprints of the dominant figure in the child's environment, that is, of the person bringing the strongest heteropsychic influence to bear upon his mind. In this way and in this way only, the term introjection assumes more than metaphorical significance. It becomes a fairly adequate description of the fact that on the mental plane total separation of parent and offspring has not as yet been accomplished and that certain attitudes emanating from figures in authority which, in our culture, take the parents' place are still operative on the *psi* level.

Similar considerations apply to the part played by the

telepathic factor in the development of the Oedipus complex. If we are justified in accepting the views held by the culturalist school we may assume that here, too, the child is apt to reflect unconscious attitudes emanating from his parents. It may derive from the son's revolt against a punitive father and culminate in his unconscious wish to usurp his place by his mother's side. This tendency may occasionally be reinforced by a frustrated mother who unconsciously seeks to use her son as a substitute lover. In a similar vein, a daughter's Oedipal attachment to her father may reflect the latter's unconscious incestuous desires toward her. Again, the child's need for sexual gratification, physical care, and attention may provoke reciprocal attitudes on the part of the significant adult and thus provide an added impetus to the development of the classical picture of the Oedipus complex.

This is not the place to go into a discussion of the vast literature dealing with this subject. The reader wishing to do so may be referred to Patrick Mullahy's[85] comprehensive survey of the field. One may either subscribe to Freud's original concepts or one may choose to follow the ideas of the Adlerian, or Jungian, or culturalist school. But in either case we must assume that a telepathic factor may play an important role also in this aspect of the child-parent relationship.

One more point may be added by way of a footnote only. It is generally assumed that the Oedipus complex makes its first appearance in the course of what Freud[44h] has described as the establishment of the child's object relationship at the age of three or four. But we have seen in the preceding chapters that there is a basic conflict in the early history of every child which precedes the development of the Oedipus complex. This conflict is constituted by his first determined efforts to assert himself as a self-contained, self-directed personality in his own right and to ward off excessive controlling influences emanating from his parents and transmitted to him on both the ego, the id, and the *psi* level. There can be no doubt that during his whole infancy he is in a state of complete and unconditional dependence on their care. Yet at the same time it is his ability to terminate this dependence and sever the ties uniting him with parental figures which is an indispensable prerequisite of his mental and emotional growth—of what C. G. Jung[65a] has described as his gradual individuation.

Many analysts have questioned the universality of the Oedipus complex. But perhaps no one will deny that there is no human being—regardless of the culture in which he is reared—whose development has not been saddled with conflicts arising from his quest for autonomy. It may well be that it is just as essential for the attainment of personality on the psychological plane as the attainment of anatomical separation by two filial cells undergoing mitosis on the physical plane. It is in view of this similarity with the birth pangs of procreation on the lowest levels of the evolutionary scale that one could describe this pre-personal, pre-genital, pre-Oedipal aspect of the struggle for individuation as the *primal conflict* of psychomitosis. Whoever has watched the relentless struggle between a possessive mother or an authoritarian father and their offspring will agree that this aspect of the child-parent relationship is of at least equal importance as its frankly sexual implications commonly described in terms of the Oedipus complex.

It is only a repetition of what should by now have become commonplace in our argument if we add at this point that all the "power operations" which are involved in the two-way struggle of the primal conflict follow the same pattern as was described in the development of fear of castration and social disapprobation as well as in the threefold stratification of parental influences which, we said, are involved in the emergence of the superego. Every individual reared in our culture is exposed to a host of influences reaching him on the ego, the id, and the *psi* level. They may either reinforce or clash with his own pregenital drives, his claims for genital satisfaction and power. It is from the subtle interaction of such three-level influences that the intricate fabric of our culture is made. They account for the way in which each individual becomes the recipient of the innumerable social clues upon which his conditioning to a given culture depends. It is three-level influences of this order which ultimately determine the prevailing mores and social attitudes approved by tradition as well as the majority of emotionally charged ideas current within a certain caste, religious denomination or professional group.

Certainly, the forces which are responsible for social and cultural integration on higher levels of the body politic are chiefly of a symbolic nature, relying on such highly differentiated means of communication as the spoken or written word and the appeal to an intellectualized code of behaviour. Disregarding the operation of the *psi* factor in the making of the vast tapestry of our contemporary Western civilization—and of all civilizations which come into our purview—would, however, be just as irrational as for fish to overlook the water in which they swim. *Psi* is a medium common to all humanity —whether or not we are aware of its existence.

These are admittedly far-reaching conclusions to draw from the limited clinical material reviewed here. Our conclusions are, however, based on data which stand for a vast number of observations of the same order. In effect, all examples of interpersonal conflict which are accessible to our primarily clinical study represent nothing but random samples of human behaviour picked from the intricate fabric of the culture in which we live.

It will be noted also that despite the shift in emphasis the majority of our conclusions is in far-reaching agreement with classical Freudian tenets. The reason is obvious. They are the result of focusing attention on essentially the same structural elements of the human mind as were originally brought out by the psychoanalytic approach. What differences emerge are largely due to the approach adopted in the present study. Psychoanalysis, applying a particular method of staining a histological slide, necessarily brings a specific type of structural detail into focus and leaves those untouched by the stain out of its frame of reference. It throws the cells that constitute the fabric of our culture into sharper relief. Our approach seeks to bring out the part played by the connecting tissue, as it were. It emphasizes the importance of the *psi* factor in its relation to the rest of the fabric of which society is made. If the total picture that emerges from doing so happens to come close to ideas held by Jung, Sullivan or E. Fromm, the present writer is only happy to acknowledge his indebtedness to them.

CHAPTER XVII

Personality Structure and Group Cohesion

HOW does our new insight into personality structure affect the picture drawn by the traditional psychoanalytic approach? In what way, if any, does it call for modification of Freud's[44d] classical description of the ego, the id, and the superego as the principal parts of the psychic apparatus? Surely, his original formulations are here to stay, much in the same way as the basic outlines of the anatomical drawings prepared by Vesalius four centuries ago have remained undisputed by subsequent generations of anatomists. Still, the development of new techniques and new tools of investigation necessitated many revisions and amplifications of his findings. Have we reached the point at which a similar revision of Freud's topographical concepts of the mind has become necessary?

According to Freud the ego is an organized part of the id, developed out of its cortical layer, as it were, and deriving its principal energies—the ego instincts—from instinctual drives originally pertaining to the id. Among the functions ascribed to the ego by psychoanalytic theory are the reception of stimuli from the outside world; the warding off of excess stimulation; control over access to motility; reality testing and storing and recall of memories. These many and varied functions have resulted in a high degree of differentiation of the ego. Psychoanalytic theory speaks of a perceptual ego, a motor ego, and so on and so forth. We have seen in Chapter XI, dealing with "Levels of Functioning and Mental Metabolism," that to this has to be added the biphasic function of anapsychic organization and catapsychic breakdown of mental content—or of the "psychic molecule"—comparable to and a direct continuation of the processes of assimilation and dissimilation on the biochemical level. We may recall, furthermore, the dual functions of empathy and enkinesis, described in Chapter XII, in which "the ego reaches out beyond its confines."

The superego is described as one of the most important subdivisions of the ego. It is derived from the child's social environment, especially from parental figures, and shows a two-fold pattern of structuralization: a vertical pattern, according to its chronological development stage by stage from infancy to adulthood, and a horizontal pattern, according to its derivation from parents and other figures in authority and from society at large.

This is not the place to go into a detailed discussion of the genetic and dynamic concepts upon which this picture has been based. I have already hinted in the preceding chapter that whatever be the part played by what Freud described as the process of identification, introjection, and incorporation in the development of the superego is undoubtedly supplemented—if not altogether determined—by heteropsychic influences impinging upon the ego. Indeed I pointed out that our assumption of a largely heteropsychic derivation of the superego places the theory of identification and introjection upon new foundations.

The part played especially by oral incorporation is common ground to psychoanalytic theory and has amply been confirmed by observations made by child analysts. Paul Schilder,[110a] describing the connection between oral incorporation and the ego's fundamental drive for mastery over its environment, specifically quotes the grasping and sucking reflex of the infant and the brain-injured patient to illustrate the deep roots of this tendency in our personality make-up. He concurs with Freud that the process of oral incorporation may result in the ego assuming some of the attitudes and mental characteristics of the introjected love object.

But how does such introjection or incorporation come about? Surely, so long as the introjection or incorporation of foodstuff is concerned the answer is obvious. But we must realize that as soon as the ego reaches out for objects that necessarily defy its attempts at actual incorporation we are merely playing with words and may easily take our own figures of speech for established facts.

Seen from our angle, Freud's concept of introjection or incorporation is, however, more than a metaphor. It is nothing but a particular phase of mental metabolism as described in Chapter XI. It is true that the formation of the superego cannot reasonably be described in terms of an actual incorporation by the child of a complete set of parental figures as a whole. What happens is the telepathic sharing of certain functionally important parental attitudes, to the exclusion of those which are indifferent within a given social context or which have no survival value to the child. Heteropsychic attitudes of this order are then subjected to the same process of catapsychic breakdown as are other influences reaching the ego from the *psi* level—or else they are assimilated by it without undergoing too far-reaching catapsychic disorganization. I emphasized that the striking similarity of mental and biochemical processes suggested by this state of affairs may well be taken as a strong argument in favour of a theory postulating the basic identity or direct continuity of the "mental" and "physical" aspects of life.

If this is true the superego can no longer be considered as a topographically well-defined and separate part of the ego nor of the individual personality structure as a whole. Derived as it is from the heteropsychic sphere it extends directly into the non-ego. It is more than a mere projection or representation of parental or other images within the ego: it amounts to their actual presence in the auto-psychic sphere, subject to their gradual assimilation by the ego. Alternatively, they may resist attempts by the ego at their assimilation and remain in a state of dissociation. We know that such split-off superego influences may then become important sources of intrapsychic conflict leading to neurotic or psychotic disorder.

The protective functions ascribed to the ego by psychoanalytic theory are fully borne out by the observations discussed in the first part of this study. Freud[440] has shown that it is the protective screen set up by the ego which helps the psychic apparatus to maintain a more or less constant level of dynamic equilibrium. Excessive stimulation both from the physical environment and from inside the body is usually conducive to anxiety. Much the same considerations apply to stimuli impinging on the ego from the heteropsychic sphere. If the influx of such stimuli remains unchecked the non-ego ceases to be a matter of indifference to the ego: it assumes a sinister, hostile character. It threatens to overwhelm the defences of the ego. Friends and relatives become sources of danger or open enemies and persecutors: the wholesale intrusion of undigested heteropsychic material into the autopsychic sphere may set off a process of schizophrenic deterioration leading to the ultimate breakdown of the personality.

The normal individual's ego defences prevent the occurrence of just this contingency. They restrict the passage of *psi* influences from "mind to mind" to an amount compatible with the individual's emotional equilibrium. The rest is subjected to the process of catapsychic disorganization, i.e., it makes its appearance in the autopsychic sphere in a symbolic disguise, distorted beyond recognition, or it is altogether repressed and fails to be registered on the conscious level.

A recent paper by Pederson-Krag[93] dealing with telepathy and repression has thrown more light upon this problem. Nevertheless, there are still vast gaps in our understanding of the dynamics of telepathic repression. We do not know why the emergence on the ego level of unconscious material from the autopsychic sphere seems to be a lesser "irregularity" in our mental organization than the occasional breakthrough of material from the *psi* level. We do not know why such an event may occasionally pass unnoticed by the person concerned while it leads to anxiety or even precipitates delusional reactions in others. The reader familiar with Jung's[65b] writings about the psychology of schizophrenia will note that a similar question in relation to the respective parts played by the individual as opposed to the collective unconscious in the pathology of schizophrenia has occupied a considerable place in the thinking of the Zurich school. The same is true for the occasional emergence of a "great dream" containing archetypal material from the collective unconscious.

Other problems affecting the psychology of the ego arise from the different ways in which various sensory or motor aspects of the ego may respond to heteropsychic influences. There undoubtedly is a visual and acoustic type prone to hallucinatory perception of optical images or spoken words, respectively. There are motor types tending to the production of so-called motor automatisms, and there are subjects whose telepathic sensitiveness is confined to occasional spells of anxiety or ill-defined bodily sensations lacking all evidence of tracer effects. All these observations are in need of further systematic investigation especially from the neuro-physiological point of view. It is from studies of this kind that a better integration of *psi* functions with our current system of neuropsychiatric thought can be expected.

A further important function of the ego is the modicum of organizing or patterning effect which it is capable of exercising upon *psi* processes, providing them with what I described as their two-faced, amphibious character. We have learned from psychoanalysis that the ego controls access to our voluntary motor functions on the one hand and to our conscious sensory impressions on the other. But we have also seen in Chapter XII that *psi* processes show a similar sensory-motor organization and that this dual organization is in turn closely related to the polarity which can be discerned in the dual functions of empathy and enkinesis (cf. Thouless and Wiesner.[129a])

Telepathy fits in well with this picture. It is an essentially two-way process aimed at extending the range of sensory-motor attitudes of the ego into the sphere of interpersonal relationships; or to be more precise: telepathy in a stricter sense is the sensory aspect of the process, while psychokinesis—that is a motor impulse directed centrifugally towards the non-ego—has to be regarded as its motor counterpart.

All these considerations make one thing perfectly clear: they indicate that the Freudian topographical picture of personality is in need of considerable modification. It has to be modified in one of two ways. According to a more conservative version the id may still be taken as the inner core of the personality structure. The ego does not, however, constitute a clearly defined and sharply circumscribed shell around it. It is potentially open to influences from both the id and *psi* in which it is immersed. In fact, it has no sharp demarcation line in either direction. In a similar vein we must assume that the superego represents but an area of specifically channelled heteropsychic influences impinging upon the ego. It is determined by both past and present experiences depending on the individual's age, family situation, and the general cultural influences to which he is exposed.

According to a more unorthodox version the ego occupies the core of the personality structure. It is responsible for its sensory-motor organization—including empathy and enkinesis—while its patterning—anapsychic and catapsychic—functions account for the appearance of the physical world and for the symbolic

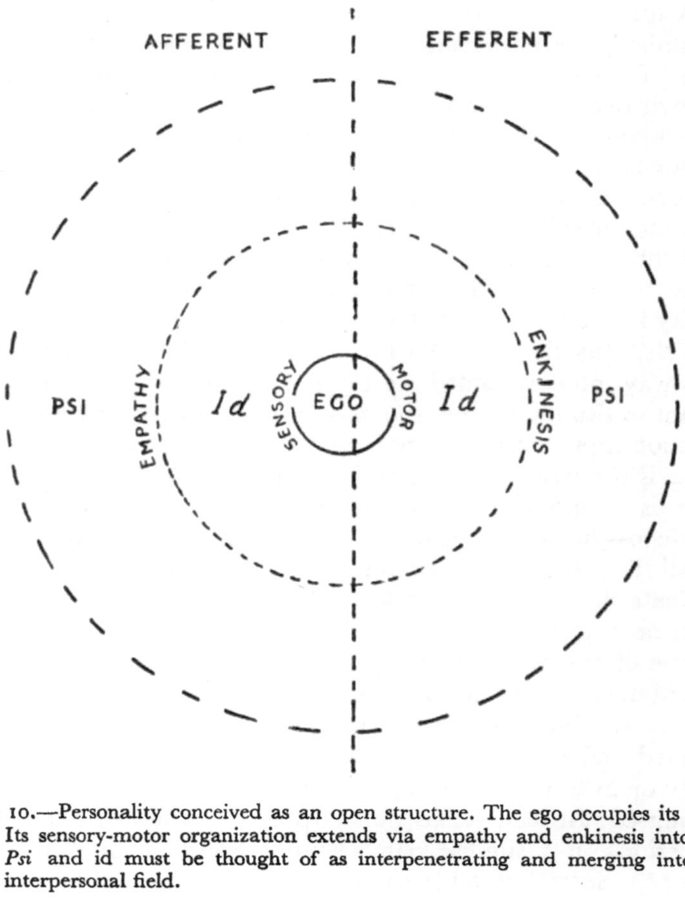

FIG. 10.—Personality conceived as an open structure. The ego occupies its core. Its sensory-motor organization extends via empathy and enkinesis into *psi*. *Psi* and id must be thought of as interpenetrating and merging into the interpersonal field.

images in which instinctual drives and occasional *psi* influences manifest themselves in consciousness (Fig. 10).

Needless to say, the sensory-motor organization of the ego extending over the area occupied by empathic and enkinetic attitudes far into the heteropsychic sphere as indicated by our diagram has to be taken with a grain of salt. We have to realize that the strict discrimination between sensory and motor functions is largely artificial even in the area of conventional ego functions. We know now that every perception involves active participation of the perceiving subject and every motor act presupposes a response to sensory stimuli and is intimately blended with the act of perception.

We must realize, furthermore, that the distinction between *psi* and id suggested by our diagram is no less artificial. We have already commented, in Chapter X, on the basically extratemporal and extraspatial characteristics common to both the id and the ego level of functioning. Both seem to require an essentially extracausal, metalogical, conceptual scheme for their better understanding. Nor are we in a position at the present stage to decide which of the two represents a more primitive or primordial stage in the scale of evolution. Indeed, the two may be nothing more than two different aspects of the same ultimate psychic reality which for obvious reasons is basically inaccessible to pictorial representation within a spatio-temporal frame of reference.

Be that as it may, the chief deviation of our concept of personality structure from the classical Freudian picture lies in the fact that it has to be considered as an open and not as a closed system. To be more precise, it is a system which may be described as open or closed, as the case may be, at various stages of a person's life history and varying as to the degree to which it is closed or open in accordance with changing functional states and life situations, particularly interpersonal relationships within a given social context. In short, personality is not a rigid immutable "structure" at all as one may be led to believe, but a living, pulsating entity expanding and contracting like a beating heart and falling in with the twenty-four-hour rhythm of rest and activity—of sleep and wakefulness in nature at large.

* * *

Personality structure conceived along these lines opens up new vistas of individual and social psychology which cannot be discussed in the present context. There is, however, one aspect of interpersonal relationships that calls for comment from our point of view: the problem of groups and group psychology.

The modern psychodynamic approach places chief emphasis upon the part played by an intricate pattern of identifications between members of a group and their leader on the one hand, and a pattern of mutual identifications taking place among members of the group on the other. In this way group cohesion is at bottom due to a libidinal bond tying group members together, comparable to the bond which exists between parent and child and the siblings among themselves. The discovery of the *psi* factor introduces a new element of group cohesion into the picture. Indeed, the evidence available so far suggests that group formation may show a wide variety of patterns according to the respective parts played by primitive instinctual drives or id factors, by *psi* processes, and by ego functions in their organization.

Proceeding from more complex and more highly differentiated forms to more primitive forms of social organization we see, first, societies of the kind represented by our own culture. Such societies are based, first and foremost, on means of social interaction and communication operating on the ego level. An intricate system of codified laws and mores governs interpersonal relationships. The democratic process has crystallized in a hierarchical scale of political, socio-economic, and financial institutions run according to more or less rational and scientifically evolved principles.

However, focusing attention on deeper levels, we become aware of the primitive, archaic elements which are involved in the operation of societies even of the highest order. We may be nothing but rational human beings when we go about our business in office, farm or factory. But when faced with the slightest deviation from our established social routine our behaviour is invariably influenced by additional factors of a non-rational nature, derived from the id level of functioning. Magic, channelized into ritualistic customs and observances, controls our responses at such biological nodal points of our lives as birth, initiation, marriage or death. Id impulses may easily get the upper hand in crowds swayed by powerful emotions.

But here, again, we have to assume that *psi* functions play an important part, especially so when action approximates the patterns of organized groups with little communication on the ego level between its members. This has been emphasized by J. Meerloo's[81a,b] recent studies of panic and group behaviour. Unfortunately, far too little is known about the operation of *psi* in groups observed in anthropological field investigations, and reports of telepathy in pre-literate tribes published in the older literature are still in need of confirmation.

Systematic experiments dealing with the same problem in the field of parapsychology proper have been few and far between. René Warcollier[135] has carried out a number of drawing tests suggesting telepathic interaction or "contagion" among those participating in the experiments. Some recent card-calling tests carried out by S. G. Soal[118a] in London were designed in such a way that two agents co-operated in transmitting two different parts of the material concerned to one of his percipients, Mrs. Stewart. These experiments, like those involving a single agent, produced highly significant results.

More recently, A. E. Buck[16] in England has paid particular attention to the problem of telepathy in group therapy. She suggests that "when a group of individuals has reached a certain minimum of *rapport* a state is then established in which a degree of telepathic interaction can occur and a particularly sensitive and constructive atmosphere is obtained."

The observations of J. L. Moreno[84] and his co-workers are highly suggestive in the same direction. However, there are no experimental data available to bear out the presumable role played by telepathy in group therapy and observations regarding spontaneous occurrences between members of such groups have only indirect bearing upon questions of therapy in general.

Yet all observations of this order—whether they be experimental or spontaneous—have one thing in common: the "groups" involved are not present "in the flesh." They are groups existing—if at all—solely on the *psi* level. There are several cases in my records which contain evidence of telepathic interaction in dreams between myself and two or three of my patients. J. Eisenbud[33e] has discussed such occurrences in his papers and Dr. Buck[16] refers to them as telepathic "inter-dreaming." However, the conditions under which this occurs are so involved and would require such detailed description of circumstances and dynamics that it would go beyond the scope of the present inquiry. Only one example of apparent collective agency with a patient of mine playing the part of the percipient may serve as an illustrative case.

The patient, Mrs. M., a woman of fifty-two, was married to a writer two years her junior. Suspecting him of marital infidelity she developed a reactive depression with suicidal ideas. Psychotherapy was at first of no avail and she received a series of electric shock treatments. Shortly after her release from hospital and following resumption of psychotherapy she had the following series of dreams which occurred during the same night.

(1) We were living in a penthouse.* Caspar and Louise came to visit us. We were serving tea.

(2) I am in Cousin Charlotta's house in D. I look at a brass tray. It is used to hold calling cards. I see a card with something written on it in Spanish.

(3) My husband and I drove to a place. It was like a hotel or a big apartment house; I showed my husband the way to drive to the front door. But he drove to a kind of parking place at the back of the house. He smiled and said: "This is the way I always drive here."

The dreams introduce a number of characters who require elucidation. Caspar and Louise are a married couple, friends of the dreamer and also of the therapist. Incidentally, it is Caspar and Louise who referred the patient to the present writer. Louise, like the patient herself, is older than her husband. Still, the marriage is successful and Caspar has never been involved with other women. They are also much better off than the dreamer and her writer husband and live in a beautiful penthouse apartment in which rather expensive

* A penthouse is an apartment—usually expensive—built on the top floor of an apartment house.

parties have been the order of the day. The patient's cousin, Charlotta, also has done much better than Mrs. M. Charlotta and her husband live in an expensive apartment house in D. with every comfort and luxury the patient could wish for herself. All this accounts for the dynamics of a substantial part of the dream material. The first two dreams express the dreamer's wish to change places with Louise on the one hand and with Charlotta on the other. Both have been more successful in their married lives than Mrs. M. It will be noted, however, that there are vast gaps left in our understanding especially of the second and third dream fragments.

Turning now to the situation on my side of the picture we see here, again, a striking correspondence in a number of details. As it happened, Louise and Caspar had been my guests on the night the patient's dreams occurred. It was the first and only occasion they had been in my house. Mrs. M., though she knew of our acquaintance, was unaware of Louise's and Caspar's visit to my house. She had never been in my private residence and knew nothing of my personal life. Nor had she been in touch with Louise and Caspar since her discharge from hospital.

Tea and sandwiches were served during the evening and the conversation revolved around two principal subjects: (1) the patient and her unhappy married life, (2) telepathy in psychoanalysis and in everyday life. Those present at the party included Mrs. Laura Dale, of the American Society for Psychical Research, and all of us contributed some personal experience in parapsychology. There was general agreement as to the reality of *psi* phenomena. Also, everybody was sorry for Mrs. M., who had made such a "mess" of her life and ruined her husband's career and tormented him with her jealousy.

There is one more detail which has to be mentioned. To their annoyance, Caspar and Louise arrived half an hour late at the party. They came by taxicab and wanted to explain to the driver how to get to their destination but the driver refused to listen. He said he knew the place well and needed no directions. As a result they had first landed at the wrong (the back) side of the apartment house on whose second floor I live. The back is occupied by garages and has a driveway in front.

On Sunday evening it is usually blocked by parked cars giving the impression of a parking lot.

Comparing the part of the dreams reviewed so far with the presumably corresponding real events it could be stated that the patient joined, as it were, in the social activities of Caspar and Louise on the one hand and of the therapist and his family on the other. To be more specific, her dreams represent a condensation (1) of Charlotta's, her cousin's, house, (2) of Caspar's and Louise's penthouse apartment and (3) of the therapist's house. At the same time it is the patient who runs the show in the dream. She is in possession of the penthouse apartment, she entertains the guests. She also seems to know better how to get to my home than the obstinate cab-driver who was in turn rolled into one person with her fumbling and ineffectual husband.

There is only one *motif* left in the dreams which has remained unexplained so far: the *motif* of the Spanish calling card lying on a brass tray, which Mrs. M. saw in her cousin's house. The patient had no associations to offer in connection with either the tray, the calling card or the Spanish words printed on it. Neither did there seem to be anything on my side of the picture which could possibly be linked up with these two items.

This gap in the understanding of the manifest dream content was so puzzling to me that I felt I had to shelve the whole incident and its suspected telepathic implications together with many other inconclusive observations of the same kind.

Three weeks later my daughter's eyes were caught by a quaint little match-box she found lying on a large copper tray on an end table in our apartment. I was not quite sure where it had come from. Then I remembered Caspar having used what I thought to be minute candle-shaped Italian matches while on his visit to our home. "They are called *Fiammiferi Italienissimi*," I explained to Barbara in a somewhat nostalgic reminiscence of pre-war travels in Italy. However, on taking another look at the box I was surprised to find that, far from being of Italian make, it hailed from Mexico. The words printed on it were in the *Spanish* language and ran as follows: "Classicos de Lujo, La Central, 90 Luces; Hecho in Mexico;

Lito-offset Latina." It also showed the manufacturer's name in bold letters: "Mendizabal Y Cia Sucs. Cia Cerillera Mexicana S.A., 4a del Pino No. 169, Mexico D.F." The face of the match-box carried a picture of the Venus of Milo and of the Parthenon in the background. Its back was adorned with a colour reproduction of Goya's *La Maja Desnuda.*

Assuming the dream is of a telepathic nature, the belated discovery of the match-box left behind by Caspar, the "caller," would well account for the *motif* of a *calling card* seen by the patient in the dream. It is true that we have to substitute copper for brass, and a rectangular article made of paper carrying the manufacturer's business address for a calling card. But this is a well-known characteristic of what I described as the telepathic scatter effect. Notwithstanding this telepathic scatter here, again, it is the combination of a number of undistorted distinctive features, common to both dream and reality, which, in conjunction with the meaningful nature of the telepathic interpretation, justifies and even calls for such a reading.

However, Mrs. M.'s dream has not been described in this connection as another case to support our thesis of the part played by telepathy in the psychoanalytic situation. It brings a new feature of the telepathic process into focus. It will be noted that while most of the presumptively telepathic elements contained in the dream had been part and parcel of my own mental contents at the time the dream occurred, this does not apply to the *motif* of the calling card and brass tray. Originally I had been utterly unaware of its very existence and later I had been mistaken in regard to the Spanish inscription on the match-box. Unless we are prepared to consider the possibility of clairvoyance or of the patient having "precognized" my belated realization of the Mexican origin of the box, this would indicate that other persons besides myself must have played the parts of telepathic agents. On inquiry I soon ascertained that my wife had indeed known from the outset all about the box. Needless to say, Caspar himself has to be credited with possessing the same information. The same has to be assumed about Louise, his wife.

Why do we dwell at such length on these trivial details? They show clearly that in this case the telepathic dream was based on information derived from more than one telepathic agent. Indeed, it may well be that it emanated from the whole group which had gathered in the present writer's apartment on the critical night. On the other hand, the patient herself seems to indicate by her dream that although she had been excluded from participating "in the flesh" in the social gathering that took place in her therapist's home, she was there nonetheless: as an unseen and uninvited guest taking mental notes of the proceedings. It will be recalled that some of the incidents observed in the cases of Fred L. and Ronald H. follow the same pattern. So does a further incident observed with Mr. H., whose case will be discussed in Chapter XXI.

In all these cases the patient's dream seemed to indicate his or her desire to participate in or to be included in a family group, thus replacing in a telepathic way the broken link with his or her own next-of-kin. Observations like these bring out an important point. They indicate that telepathy, besides being a factor potentially involved on all levels of interpersonal relationships, may occasionally be the only link existing between two or more individuals separated from each other in space. Telepathy may thus constitute a more or less autonomous factor, however tenuous, responsible for group formation.

However, our example demonstrates at the same time the extremely loose, indeed rudimentary, organization of groups whose existence is confined to the *psi* level only. While members of groups operating on the id level may be cognizant at least of the physical presence of their fellows swayed by the same collective emotions of panic, rage or enthusiasm, none of those contributing to the telepathic dreams described here—including the dreamer herself—was in any way aware of his or her membership in a group. Nor did the fleeting moment that marked a "meeting of their minds" have any appreciable effect upon whatever bonds of friendship had existed between them before. Mrs. M.'s condition failed to improve and she had again to seek admission to a hospital. Louise and Caspar have remained unaware until now of their brief involvement in the telepathic incident described. Mrs. Dale learned of it only at the time of writing this and helped to reconstruct details referring to the evening from her own recollection.

Summing up, it can be stated that the integration of groups, in order to be effective, must embrace three levels. *Tres faciunt collegium*. It is as though the integration of three levels of personality structure were needed for the formation and effective functioning of groups. Under primitive conditions group cohesion may remain confined to the id level. We all are made of the same stuff, derived, psychologically speaking, from the id. Closely knit family groups, clans, and kinships illustrate the point. But the connecting link between their members may in part be supplied by the *psi* level. This is particularly true for so-called spiritualistic development circles, religious groups and well-integrated therapy groups. The best example of effective three-level integration, although without conscious reference to *psi* factors, may be represented by participants in such spontaneous group activities as Moreno's psychodrama.[84] By contrast, group coherence under what is usually considered as civilized conditions is largely confined to ego levels only. Such collectives may be highly articulate and have the most ingenious tools of technical communication at their disposal. However, in the absence of deeper psychological bonds they remain poorly integrated and their function as a group problematical. At the time of writing the similarity of such organizations with the UN does not seem to be merely coincidental.

CHAPTER XVIII

Telepathy and Cerebral Localization

IT seems to be a characteristic feature of every culture that some of its basic, pre-scientific concepts are tacitly taken for granted and exempt from the process of gradual restatement and readjustment to new insight gained by the increase of scientific knowledge. Our concepts of mind and body and their assumed inter-relationship belong to this category.

Whether we consider mind and body as two fundamentally different entities, or regard one as a mere reflection or epiphenomenon of the other, whether we hold with Bishop Berkeley that our perceptual world is the only absolute reality, or follow the lead of the behaviourists and place our reliance on the reality of the material world, our language remains committed to the traditional dualistic philosophy which has come down to us from classical antiquity and from the early and medieval Christian era.

This attitude is not confined to our thinking on the level of common sense—to what the philosophers describe as the naïve realism of the man in the street. It is also contained in the reasoning of the biologist, the physiologist, and the neurologist. Certainly, the authors of our modern textbooks of neurology would resolutely protest against any continued adherence to such unwarranted, pre-scientific concepts. Yet however materialistic, Pavlovian or behaviouristic their orientation may be, they can hardly avoid using the nomenclature of a past voluntaristic school of psychology which takes volition and the purposive nature of man's actions for granted and which describes the clenching of my fist as a spontaneous motor act by contrast to the blinking of my eye which is described as an "involuntary" reflex action.

It is true that this manner of speaking can be replaced by a cumbersome system of circumlocutions which carefully avoids the use of introspective psychological terms. Still, common sense will always insist that the actions of my muscular system can be willed, whereas the functions of my inner organs are independent of conscious control. Indeed, the clinical neurologist, whatever his philosophical leanings, tacitly accepts this principle when he describes the functions of the upper motor neuron as *voluntary* or spontaneous and ascribes the ability to transmit perceptions to the brain cortex to afferent, *sensory* neurons. In fact, the postulate of a motor and sensory region in the brain cortex, located in the anterior and posterior central convolution respectively, is one of the cornerstones of neurophysiology.

Experimental and clinical research into the localization of such specialized functions as speech, reading, writing, etc., essentially follows the same dual pattern of inquiry into motor and sensory aspects. Among its achievements it can claim the discovery of the centres of Broca and Wernicke and the identification of an area in the left angular gyrus the lesion of which results in Gerstman's[49] finger agnosia, agraphia, and acalculia. More modern work on cortical localization of a rather precise nature is summarized in the textbooks of physiological psychology and need not be reviewed here.

However, despite the great strides made by cerebral localization, recent advances of clinical neurology dashed the hope of ultimately arriving at a flawless map charting all the known functions of the organism on the brain surface. Modern Gestalt psychology undermined the atomistic concept of mental activity upon which the doctrine of strictly specialized punctiform cerebral localization is based and a new school of neurological thinking influenced by Henry Head,[54] Kurt Goldstein[51] and their co-workers, is inclined to reject altogether the theory of a fixed structural basis for every given act, motor or sensory.

It is in the light of these general considerations that we have to approach the question with which we are concerned in this chapter: the question of the cerebral localization of telepathy and *psi* functions in general. In trying to do so we have to bear in mind the limitations of our established knowledge regarding cortical localization to which we have pointed just before. We have to realize that our attitude towards all problems involving the so-called mind-body relationship is beset by a conflicting attitude inherent in our cultural heritage. On the one hand we have been conditioned by the structure of our language to think of mind and matter as two disparate entities, one attached to the other in some unaccountable way. On the other hand we are cautioned by the physiologist as the spokesman of modern materialistic science against the use of these debatable concepts in a strictly scientific inquiry. The behaviourist psychology school especially advises us to evaluate all available neuro-physiological data without reference to such purely introspective terms as consciousness, free will, sensory experience, and the like.

Yet the fact is that the physiologist himself does not always adhere to his own precepts. He may be contented with studying the chain of physical events set into motion when a ray of light strikes our retina. He continues by recording the electric, electro-physiologic or muscular responses elicited in the organism and he can pride himself with having arrived at a fairly complete picture of all the processes intervening between stimulus and response. However, it is also true to say that when he takes time off from his laboratory he cannot help becoming aware of the gap which exists, so far as his own inner experience is concerned, between stimulus and response. He knows that whatever chemical or physiological changes occur in his sense organs, in his brain, and in his muscular system, he is also aware of sounds, colours, and memory images or other subjective experiences which are evoked by them. He is used to considering this "non-inferential" knowledge as mental, by contrast to his "inferential" knowledge of the outer world which he considers as physical. He also knows that there is a gap between the two. But he has become used to glossing over its existence: for the simple reason that it does not seem to make any difference to the validity of objective findings made in his particular field of research.

I indicated, however, that it is just when he is called upon to deal with the question of cerebral localization that he cannot avoid coming face to face with the gap intervening between stimulus and response. He may be perfectly satisfied that a visual impression is brought about by electronic or molecular changes, transmitted along certain neural pathways to the lateral geniculate body and the calcarine fissure of the brain cortex. But he is at a loss to tell in what way, if any, electronic or molecular changes are transformed into the perception of the colour red or the emotion of happiness or grief.

He may have learned from Bertrand Russell[108] that "sensation is the first mental effect of a cause" and that "volition is the last mental cause of a physical effect," but he cannot establish the nature of the tenuous link between the two. In short, he is ignorant of the way in which to quote Bertrand Russell again, "matter affects mind in sensation and mind affects matter in volition."

Now he may well assert that this is a problem of no scientific importance. To quote a well-known adage: "What is mind? No matter. What is matter? Never mind." However, in discussing the presumable anatomical basis of the telepathic process such a supercilious attitude is no longer tenable. One cannot brush aside the problem of how autopsychic awareness comes about, yet demand at the same time a satisfactory explanation of the *modus operandi* of heteropsychic awareness. Again, whatever answer can be offered to the latter question, it is obvious that it must contain references to difficulties encountered in dealing with the former. Indeed, in seeking to find an anatomical basis for telepathy our difficulties are augmented by the very fact of its "extrasensory" nature. We have seen in Chapter IX that *psi* functions are hard to reconcile with our classical space-time scheme of thinking. We know that a vast number of laboratory experiments, some of them carried out over thousands of miles, show that the operation of ESP is independent of distances involved. Telepathy is thus in flagrant contradiction to the established laws of radiation. There is no known form of energy which can conceivably be held responsible for the transmission of a telepathic impression. Worse still, we know of no sense organ or other anatomical substratum which could conceivably be the basis for its reception nor of any pathway, neural or humoral, to carry it to our cortical centres.

In what way, if any, are we then capable of catching an occasional telepathic glimpse of another person's mental content? What is the physiological basis of heteropsychic sensitiveness and what are the means by which transmission of volitional impulses from "mind to mind" may become effective? There seems to be only one way to deal with this baffling question. We have to throw overboard our traditional —yet scientifically unwarranted—concepts regarding cerebral localization, and the mind-body relationship in general, and replace it by a new concept which is in better keeping with both the old and the newly established facts.

What is the principal tenet of the old, time-honoured doctrine of mind-body relationship? It is the belief that all my inner experiences—my perceptual images, feelings, thoughts and volitional impulses—are strictly private and confined to my own brain or central nervous system. Obviously, this doctrine has to be abandoned so as to make allowance for the fact that some of my private experiences may become "public" some of the time "without the aid of the familiar channels of sensation." In short, we have to give up the idea of a punctiform, ego-centric, uni-cerebral localization of "consciousness" and adopt the theory of a potential *multi-cerebral* or *scattered* localization of mental processes. To put it in other words: we have to conceive of human personality in terms of a potentially open system as described in the previous chapter, or rather of a personality field sweeping across the boundary lines of strictly isolated individual units.

We had already reached this conclusion when we discussed the psychodynamics of the telepathic process. But the question is whether the formulation suggested here can really be taken for an answer to our problem. It can be argued that our thesis is little more than a mere elaboration of the fact of heteropsychic experience, in contradistinction to what we described as autopsychic experience. We may be told that our formulation still leaves us in the dark as to the way in which we become aware of heteropsychic experiences. But we have to realize at this point that we are faced with the identical difficulty when we try to answer the same question in regard to the autopsychic sphere. We have seen that here, too, the gap between brain event and inner experience is difficult to bridge. Even reference to the fact that in ordinary experience sensory stimuli are conducted along familiar neural pathways is beside the point. Conscious experience within the autopsychic sphere is possible without the intervention of afferent neural pathways of conduction. This is true for the majority of thought processes; for hallucinations and for our dream life. Indeed, the absence of afferent conducting pathways involved in our inner experience is a characteristic which telepathy and hallucinations have in common. Both illustrate the disconnection between "mental" and "physical" in a striking manner.

Professor C. E. M. Joad,[64] rendering a passage from my book *Telepathy and Medical Psychology*[32] in his own words, put it as follows: "We have not the faintest idea how the transition from event in the brain to experience in consciousness is effected. Hence the fact that there is an unbridgeable gulf in our knowledge of the mode by which what is going on in one mind is communicated to another is not so odd as it at first might appear. There is an equally unbridgeable gap in our knowledge of the mode by which what is going on in the body and brain is communicated to the mind that animates them. We forget the mystery of the latter only because it is common; we are astonished by the oddness of the former only because it is rare."

The materialistic philosopher or behaviourist psychologist will probably be dissatisfied with such a formulation. To him any inquiry into the physical basis of conscious experience is meaningless. Strictly speaking he should therefore not be concerned at all with the problem of cerebral localization of telepathy either, involving as it does a certain aspect of our inner experience described as heteropsychic. But if this is so he cannot legitimately demand an answer to a question which, according to his own premises, is meaningless. The fact is that heteropsychic awareness involves the same baffling problem of consciousness as autopsychic awareness, even though in the former instance it is magnified by the vastly greater spatial extension of the gap between "mental" and "physical."

What, then, is the relevance of our formulation to the broader problems of neuro-physiology and cerebral localization? What is the heuristic value of the theory of a potential pluri-cerebral localization of consciousness as proposed here, viewed against the background of our current knowledge about the mind-body relationship? We will presently see that its chief—perhaps its only—merit lies in the fact that it is in better keeping with *all* the available data referring to the mind-body relationship than the classical theory of uni-cerebral localization of mental processes within the confines of personality conceived as a detached, isolated, and closed system.

The salient facts concerning cerebral localization within the autopsychic sphere can briefly be summarized as follows. There is a hierarchical scale of precision with which each sensory stimulus reaching us from the outer world or from the inside of our body is registered in our consciousness. The accuracy of our visual or tactile or kinesthetic perception can be said to top the scale, even though there are marked differences in the accuracy of our eyesight, e.g. between the focal and peripheral regions of the retina. Sensations from our inner organs are much more indistinct and usually lacking in local signs. As a general rule we are altogether unaware of our heartbeat and know nothing of the existence of our appendix —at least as long as it is not inflamed. Whether our hair, nails or clothing are still to be considered as parts of our ego or body scheme may be a matter of controversy.

The same hierarchical scale can be discerned in turning to motor aspects of the autopsychic sphere. The skilled movements of our eye muscles, fingers, hands, vocal chords, etc., can be effected with a high degree of accuracy. The muscles of our forehead, of our toes or our torso lack the same capacity of strictly selective innervation. Spontaneous actions channelized into these areas of our muscular system result in more loosely co-ordinated associated or synkinetic movements. Again, no one can innervate his heart muscle at will. Finally, the movements of our intestinal tract are equally as inaccessible to spontaneous volition as a limb paralysed by organic lesion or by a process of hysteric conversion. Motor paralysis and anaesthesia, organic or functional, may altogether remove the affected part from the autopsychic sphere, even though its anatomical continuity with the body may be preserved. Put in terms of Freud's ego psychology one could say that, under normal circumstances, movements of our fingers, hands or lips are closer to the ego than those of the muscles of the trunk or of our left little toe, and that a paralysed leg may be still further removed from our ego. Passing from the autopsychic to the heteropsychic sphere it is readily understood that the bodies of our fellow-men, like the rest of the world, are outside of our ego and usually described as non-ego. As a general rule we are not prepared to consider even the remote possibility of extending our volitional control to their muscular system or of reaching out to some aspect of their private sensory experience as though it were our own.

However, such occasional heteropsychic effects of our tendency to vicarious functioning or enkinesis and emphatic response as were discussed in preceding chapters make a thorough revision of the traditional theory of punctiform, uni-cerebral localization of both will and sensation necessary.

The classical cerebro-centric or uni-cerebral concept of the mind-body relationship remains true—within limitations. For all practical intents and purposes, my brain is in exclusive control of my, and only my, sensory-motor responses. However, under special conditions my volitional impulse may have an observable effect upon another person's motor behaviour. In the same vein, under special circumstances, there is a telepathic element involved in my empathic response to the thoughts, feelings or to the sum total of another person's mental content. Such heteropsychic implications of my behaviour, motor or sensory, may be few and far between. In effect the odds against them increase more and more as we move further away from the imaginary co-ordinate of the ego as shown on the chart on page 216.

Figuratively speaking, the efficacy of my volitional impulse to move my right index finger may be put at 100 per cent. It may be only 50 per cent when I try to raise my left eyebrow. It may be close to zero when a hemiplegic patient seeks to lift his paralysed leg—and the odds against success of my effort to induce a percipient seated in the room next door to do the same thing may be astronomical. Nevertheless, the famous Brugmans–Van Dam[15] experiment in which the experimenter

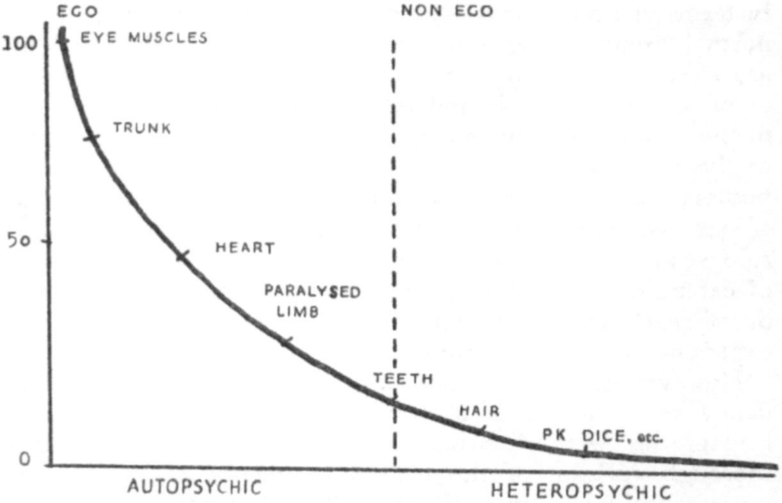

FIG. 11.—The graph shows the diminishing effect of volitional effort as we proceed from the ego to the non-ego, from the autopsychic to the heteropsychic sphere. An identical graph would express the same state of affairs in relation to sensory experiences. The diagrammatic concept of psycho-physical parallelism applies only to the area very close to the ego. Beyond that the relationship amounts to a psycho-physical gradient as illustrated by the curve.

tried to make the subject's hand move to a certain square on a draughtboard one floor below shows that under certain circumstances precisely this may be possible to achieve. More than that, if we are prepared to accept the validity of Dr. Rhine's still controversial dice-throwing experiments, we would have to consider the possibility of psychokinesis, i.e. of a direct impact of volition upon things in the physical world. We know that, likewise, the acuity of sensory perception drops steeply as we proceed from the autopsychic to the heteropsychic sphere —from the ego to the non-ego. But Dr. Rhine's[103c] ESP experiments under so-called clairvoyant conditions indicate that here, too, we may be able to score in excess of chance expectation even on such indifferent, ego-alien material as the Zener cards.

From a purely pragmatic point of view the mind-body relationship can thus best be represented by an asymptotic curve plotting the efficacy of voluntary action (or the accuracy of sensory perception) on the vertical, and the distance from the imaginary position of the ego on the horizontal co-ordinate.

Certainly, our diagram cannot be substantiated by reference to strictly quantitative data. But even so it should go far to show that the concept of psycho-physical parallelism upon which so many of our neuro-physiological premises are based (and which also is little else than a diagrammatic concept) cannot possibly give justice to the facts as they appear in the marginal zones of the autopsychic sphere. It has to be replaced by what might be described as the concept of a psycho-physical *gradient*, extending from the ego to the non-ego and thereby eliminating the strict boundaries between the two.

Despite the gap involved in this, as in any other, concept of the assumed mind-body relationship this formulation in any case holds the advantage of fitting the facts of telepathy and related phenomena within a scientifically consistent scheme of neuro-physiology and of doing so in a way which is at least as consistent as the time-honoured classical scheme of cerebral localization. It has, moreover, the added advantage of saving us the embarrassment of having to relegate *psi* phenomena into a scientific no-man's-land of the occult or mystical.

There is no denying that the concept of multi-cerebral localization and of a psycho-physical gradient as proposed here still carries the marks of the traditional dualistic approach and therefore falls short of an ultimately desirable unified theory of psychology. But we may recall that the same is true for virtually all formulations at present used in the field proper of neuro-physiology. It may well be that both the classical and the present approach to the problem of cerebral localization—uni-cerebral or otherwise—would be better off if they could rid themselves from the shackles of our time-honoured dualistic thinking. This, however, is an objective which goes beyond the scope of our inquiry. We must be satisfied in the present context with noting that, according to current theory, the quality of consciousness is attached in some unaccountable way to the confines of one, and only one person's brain substance. Or as Bertrand Russell[108] puts it, "each region of the brain is a class of events and among the class of events constituting a region thoughts are included." Our formulation amplifies this statement and enables us to make allowance for the fact that the quality of consciousness may be attached to loosely knit clusters of "brain regions" scattered in space and lacking the continuity or fixed anatomical integrity of one individual brain.

The question of what "brain regions" are specifically concerned with telepathic experiences is of secondary importance. Their vagueness and poor organization are reminiscent of so-called *protopathic* sensations usually connected with thalamic centres. Again, the absence of volitional control characteristic of both *psi* functions and extra-pyramidal muscular action points to the basal ganglia as the areas which may play a part in the motor aspect of the telepathic process. It should also be recalled that both telepathy and extra-pyramidal activities can be mobilized by strong motivations under the influence of affect. We have to realize, furthermore, that neither *psi* functions nor the functions of the extra-pyramidal or thalamic centres can be strictly separated from sensory or motor functions of a more highly organized, epicritic nature. We know that impulses generated in thalamic centres are involved in every sensory impression. In the same way motor impulses originating in the extra-pyramidal system are an integral part of every motor act carried out under the control of the higher cortical centres.

Such specific neurological considerations as these should not, however, obscure the fact that our current conceptual scheme of cerebral localization has no room for *psi* functions. We have emphasized that their very existence can only be reconciled with a new conceptual scheme based on the concept of a *psychophysical gradient* and a potential *pluri-cerebral* localization of mental processes. And we shall see in the chapter that follows that this concept calls in turn for a new scientific scheme of thinking, transgressing the boundary lines of time, space, and causality: for what can be described as a *metalogical* frame of reference.

There is another argument that can be invoked in support of our thesis. Anybody who has cast a glance on a bacterial culture in a microscope; on a deposit of spawn on the surface of a pond; or on the teeming crowd of an insect heap knows that life itself has the tendency to be scattered through the universe in spatio-temporal clusters. Yet despite the absence of fixed anatomical structures responsible for their integration such clusters can be observed to operate as coherent and organized wholes. We hinted in Chapter XIII that the same is true for the sequence of successive filial generations constituting the developmental profile of an animal species. Here, too, the lawful operation of certain integrated overall patterns of behaviour can be discerned. They are usually ascribed to hereditary transmission of structural and functional characteristics. But here, too, as in the case of cerebral localization, the geneticist is hard put to it when he tries to put his finger on the anatomical substratum in which he assumes all the host of hereditary traits and potentialities of an organism are anchored. He may be told by the physicist that it is a miniature atomic code script compressed into the nucleus of a fertilized egg from which the whole future development of the organism is to evolve (Schroedinger).[113] But is not this link connecting the successive generations of a species in the perspective of time just as tenuous as the fleeting telepathic link connecting two individuals of a species scattered in space? It appears that at this point the temporal and the spatial aspects of the biological identity of a species can no longer be separated. Its historical or biological identity, safeguarded by hereditary transmission of traits, seems to merge with its solidarity in the perspective of space borne out by the potential interaction between members of a species on the *psi* level. It may well be that it is precisely the genetic link between past, present, and future of a species which is also responsible for the occasional "meeting of the minds" of individuals scattered in space yet retrieving lost vestiges of their original unity in an occasional flash of telepathic communication.

PART THREE

CAN IT BE APPLIED IN PRACTICE?

AN APPROACH TO THERAPY

If you consider the individual by himself, then you see of man just as much as you see of the moon; only man with man provides a full image.

MARTIN BUBER, *Between Man and Man*

CHAPTER XIX

The Psychotherapist Takes His Bearings

MODERN psychotherapy aims at influencing human behaviour by means of rational techniques evolved and tested according to established scientific principles. In its traditional form it seeks to help the individual to attain a richer life compatible with existing social standards. The basic orientation of modern psychotherapy is thus first and foremost scientific. It considers human personality as a closed system of instinctual drives modified by the impact of its social and physical environment but subject to the same laws of cause and effect which govern the universe at large.

It is true that there is no school of psychotherapy, psychoanalytic or otherwise, which has tried to uphold such an uncompromisingly materialistic approach in a consistent way. Paul Schilder,[110a] Jules Masserman[78], Franz Alexander,[3] to quote only a few protagonists of modern dynamic psychiatry, consider psychotherapy both a science and an art. Far from confining their inquiry to purely causal or etiological aspects, they stress the importance of the patient's goals and motivations. In short, they make due allowance for the apparent purposefulness of human behaviour: for what philosophers call its teleological aspects.

From a strictly materialistic point of view there is a striking inconsistency in such a position although, by tacit agreement, as it were, we are in the habit of disregarding its existence. Like our notions of the dichotomy of body and mind it has become part and parcel of our cultural heritage. We are satisfied that our body consists of the same elementary particles as the rest of the world. We conceive of its functions in terms of a mechanistic series which can fully be accounted for by well-known biochemical and electrophysiological processes. Yet at the same time we cling to the belief in the spontaneity of our actions and in the independence of our goals and motivations from the laws of cause and effect. That is, we think of our behaviour as part of a teleological series, purposeful, free, and goal directed.

It is true that the astronomer, the chemical engineer or even the manufacturer of television sets can go about his business without being unduly concerned over the inconsistency of his general outlook on the world—his *Weltanschauung*. But this inconsistency is brought into sharper focus whenever we approach the problem of human behaviour in health and disease in a truly scientific spirit. The physician, brought up in the materialistic or monistic tradition of the turn of the century, may easily be led to thinking of disease, mental or physical, in terms of nothing but cause and effect. Yet in his daily practice, when dealing with people and their afflictions, he is compelled to make allowance for their goals and motivations, that is, to think in terms of a non-mechanistic, teleological series which does not easily fit in with his materialistic frame of reference. He may feel that he has overcome the dualistic fallacy of bygone days implied in the distinction between the organic and functional, but he finds to his surprise that, while banishing the problem from clinic and research laboratory, it is still there in his waiting room, demanding appropriate action. This is obviously due to the latent dichotomy inherent even in the modern psychosomatic approach—although we are in the habit of disregarding or glossing over its existence.

Alexander and French,[3] in their *Studies in Psychosomatic Medicine*, rightly speak of the dual personality of the old-time medical practitioner. Alexander seeks to overcome this personality split by resorting to what the history of philosophy is wont to describe as the double-aspect theory of the mind-body relationship, or the doctrine that the two are head and tail of the same penny, as it were, the one accessible to exploration from outside, by physical methods, the other revealing itself to our inner, subjective experience only and, therefore, requiring inquiry from the psychological angle. Most workers in modern psychosomatic medicine have assumed basically the same position.

Does this formulation do away with the dichotomy of two conflicting methods of investigation? The careful study of recent contributions to psychosomatic medicine reveals that this is not the case. It appears that whatever be the philosophical orientation of the respective investigator, he cannot escape the dilemma of dealing with his subject in terms of either a mechanistic or a teleological series. Professor Gardner Murphy,[86b] in his *Historical Introduction to Modern Psychology*, sums up this state of affairs when he writes: "One might expect from such studies renewed effort at some sort of rational formulation of functional mind-body interdependence, if not some high-flying philosophical solution of the mind-body problem. Actually, however, no such happy consummation can be noticed."

Yet psychiatrists and psychotherapists of the past decades have been keenly aware of the basic unity of human personality. They may have been forced to avail themselves of one-sided and often inconsistent methods of approach. Their theories may have emphasized causal or teleological aspects, as the case may be. But even though they failed to integrate their therapeutic actions within a scientifically consistent system of thought, they learned to shift their emphasis from "functional" to "organic" aspects to answer existing needs in a pragmatic manner.

One of Freud's great contributions to contemporary dynamic psychiatry is his discovery of the basically goal-directed, and therefore purposeful, nature of the neurotic symptom. But at the same time he emphasized the deterministic nature of mental processes, subject to the same laws of cause and effect as apply to the physical world. By contrast, the Adlerian school of thought based its approach on the concept of freedom and purpose as the master-key to the understanding of behaviour in both health and disease. Paul Schilder,[110b] Erich Fromm,[46] and more recently Thomas French[43] have duly acknowledged the justification of this attitude. Again, Otto Rank's[97] method of Will Therapy moves along explicitly teleological, indeterministic lines. Likewise, Wilhelm Reich's[100] technique of character analysis made important concessions to the teleological approach especially in his emphasis on the patient's character defences, while A. Kardiner[68a] specifically emphasizes the defensive and protective purpose of the patient's "intrapsychic manœuvres." C. G. Jung,[65] devoting a special philosophical study to the dichotomy of causal versus teleological inquiry in psychoanalysis, arrived at the conclusion that both have to be considered as legitimate methods of psychotherapeutic theory and practice.

More recent studies of so-called teleological mechanisms,[41] feed-back systems, etc., hold out the hope that the age-old polarity of body and mind, of organic and functional will ultimately be resolved. J. Ruesch's and G. Bateson's[107] brilliant exposition of the theory of communication applied to human affairs seems to be an important step in this direction. But whether the new science of cybernetics is capable of bridging the gap which separates an electronic computer, however complex and ingenious, from a human brain is another question. In any case, the human brain contemplating its own accomplishments is still reluctant to attribute the same capacity of contemplation to the man-made machine, and even the scientist ready to discard belief in freedom and purpose as an illusion will admit that clinging to such an illusion is one important point of difference between man and his prodigious brain child: the electronic computer device.

Be that as it may, the main contrast between the medical practitioner of a past era and the modern psychodynamic approach consists in the fact that while the former has chiefly been interested in the causes of a given sign or symptom, the latter is equally concerned with its cause and its purpose as seen against the background of the patient's motivations as a total personality. Four simple examples taken from the field of psychosomatic medicine may illustrate the point.

A patient develops diarrhoea, fever, and a fleeting erythematous rash on his abdomen. Bacteriological and serological studies reveal B. typhosum as the etiological organism. Thus the cause of his disease is ascertained and the course of therapeutic action is determined. At night the patient becomes delirious and seems to be engaged in some purposeful activity such as picking breadcrumbs from his bed-sheet. Obviously, in this case the etiological inquiry deserves our principal attention and the question of purpose of his delirious behaviour is negligible.

Another patient develops a common cold due to virus infection. Here, too, our therapeutic action is determined by the existing etiology. Yet closer examination may reveal that he has been in the habit of contracting common colds whenever he was faced with threatening life situations. This arouses the suspicion of a partly "diplomatic" nature of his illness and may give an important clue as to his treatment.

A third patient, a divorced woman of twenty-eight, became violently ill and vomited after excessive alcohol consumption. Her condition appeared so serious to the referring physician that she was admitted to a surgical ward. Psychosomatic investigation showed that her illness was of functional origin. In addition to its being due to alcoholic indulgence, it followed an attempt on the same night by her ex-husband to resume marital relations with her. Unable as she was to cope with sex on a mature level, her gastrointestinal symptoms expressed her aggressive tendencies towards her ex-husband and her disgust at his sexual practices. At the same time they were an effective means to keep him at arm's length from her. This, at bottom, teleological interpretation gave a satisfactory account of the psychodynamics of her reaction. When the interpretation was offered to the patient the presenting symptoms disappeared.

Personality study in a fourth patient, a man of fifty-two years, who suffered from bronchial asthma, revealed significant psychological factors involved in his condition. His attacks could well be considered equivalents of crying in a person whose life history had been nothing but a series of continued frustrations. Skin tests revealed no significant allergies; his asthma had been long-standing. There were fibrotic changes in the lungs and evidence of cardiovascular sclerosis. Psychotherapy was ineffective in this patient, he responded to aminophyllin injections given during the attack.

In all these cases inquiry into the cause of the existing pathology certainly is of primary importance. But the finding of B. typhosum in the first patient is obviously of greater significance than the part played by alcoholic indulgence in our third patient. In any case, the proper understanding of the psychodynamics of her symptom—of its purpose and meaning—gave the key to her therapeutic management. Again, in view of the structural changes that had developed in the fourth patient, the limitations of a one-sided psychological approach were obvious.

These four examples, commonplace though they are, show that giving mere lip-service to the dual aspect presented by all psychosomatic pathology is not enough; a flexible, double-barrelled diagnostic and therapeutic approach is required. It calls for a therapist capable of switching his focus of attention any time from a mechanistic to a teleological frame of reference, and *vice versa*, always on guard against being caught in the one to the exclusion of the other.

Specifically, the psychotherapeutic approach is concerned with the purpose and meaning of an existing functional disturbance. Unless the psychotherapist subscribes to an extreme materialistic or behaviouristic school of thought he looks at it as an expression of the patient's motivations, conscious or unconscious, and seeks to modify and readjust his neurotic reactions by making use of the clues obtained from the proper understanding of his meaningful behaviour. Behaviourists and neo-behaviourists have pointed out that references to goals and purposes are merely "abbreviations" to express a highly complicated state of affairs in which such words have to be replaced by statements about "operant conditioning," the "law of effect" and the like (B. F. Skinner[117]). But using the abbreviations evolved by the habit of teleological thinking is an invaluable short cut towards a better understanding of virtually all manifestations of personality on both the verbal and non-verbal level. Indeed, dispensing with them would be just as unreasonable as for the mathematician to refrain from availing himself of the aid of algebraic symbols and to confine himself, in the interest of science, to elementary arithmetics.

A chess player's moves may be fully accounted for in behaviourist or mechanistic terms by a "present push" in conjunction with the effect of what C. K. Kluckhohn and H. A. Murray[69] have described as "serial goal images." Yet such a description gives justice to one aspect of his behaviour only. It can be stated that a person's verbal behaviour is due to nothing but an intricate series of neuro-muscular reflexes. Yet we cannot overlook that at the same time it conveys meaning to another person. The same is true for a sign or symptom in psychosomatic medicine—even though it developed without any conscious intention on the part of the patient. In the case of our patient suffering from typhoid fever his elevated temperature is exclusively part of a mechanistic series, as is, to a lesser degree, his picking imaginary crumbs from the bed-sheet, since this is also amenable to a quasi-teleological interpretation. Again, the physician of our conversion hysteric who failed to understand the meaning and purpose of her vomiting entirely missed the point when viewing her case within an exclusively mechanistic frame of reference.

Franz Alexander[3a] has pointed out that the more direct is the relationship of affected structures to the voluntary nervous system, that is, to the cerebral cortex, the more explicit is their meaningful nature. Reverting to our diagram charting what we described as the psychophysical gradient, one could say that the closer an event to the vantage point of the ego the more compelling is its teleological interpretation to the naïve observer.

On the other side of the scale are structural lesions of the body or physical changes in the universe at large. It goes without saying that on approaching this end of the scale interpretation in terms of meaning and purpose becomes less and less applicable. In any case events in what is usually described as the physical sphere can well be accounted for within a purely mechanistic frame of reference, without regard to teleological aspects. This applies to such widely divergent happenings as the fracture of a bone, the decay of a tooth or to the falling of rocks on the mountain side—although it is true that in the former case the element of accident proneness with all its implications may enter the picture—to say nothing of the wary mountaineer who may be led to mistake a haphazard configuration of rocks for a meaningful trail-marking showing the way to the nearest shelter. (Obviously, in this instance the sole criterion in deciding whether or not meaning is attached to his ambiguous signpost is by finding out whether it was made by human hands.)

Much the same considerations apply when we are dealing with such manifestations as language, organ-language or the psychosomatic symptom. Accidental pressure applied to the chest of a dead body laid out in the morgue may result in air passing through its larynx. Yet only in the living are we justified in describing this physical event as a sign of anguish or despair. More pertinent is the interpretation of an epileptic seizure in terms of violent abreaction of hostility on an unconscious level.

In fact, when we are confronted with "behaviour" in its broadest sense psychological interpretation is inescapable. It is a natural consequence of the human situation that the functional state of a person's organs and organ-systems conveys messages to his fellow. His motor, vasomotor, and glandular reactions, voluntary and involuntary, assume the significance of expressive movements arousing fear, disgust, sympathy, and sexual excitement, as the case may be. The function of his speech muscles has specialized in this direction. They are generally considered as *the* organs of expression and communication. But the fact is that the functional state of other organs may serve the same purpose even though in a very imperfect way. The whimper of the hungry infant is a case in point. Again, the bedwetting problem-child, protesting against the lack of parental affection, is an example of conveying meaning obscured by its unintentional and equivocal nature. There were indications in the analysis of our hysteric patient that on a deeper level her vomiting expressed both her fear of being, and her desire to be, pregnant.

Language and organ-language, as studied by psychosomatic medicine, have one thing in common: they convey meaning "to whom it may concern"; the former to one's fellow-men, to one's social environment; the latter to the medical psychologist who possesses the key to its translation into ordinary language. The language of the organs is largely symbolic, like the language of the dream. Its syntax is rudimentary, its logic confused and self-contradictory. But it is derived from powerful drives, it expresses needs that urgently call for gratification and it may do so with the obstinacy of the infant crying for his bottle.

It is obviously this close relationship of disturbed organ

function to repetitive expressive movements (and the attending need to be understood by one's fellows) which accounts for at least part of the therapeutic effect of psychoanalytic interpretation in these cases. Once the patient is satisfied that the message contained in his expressive movements (or in the coded language of a functionally diseased organ) has reached a sympathetic ear he is less in need of the tedious repetition of the message called symptom.

* * *

How does telepathy—and how do *psi* functions in general—fit into this picture? We have seen in Chapter X that the laws governing the *psi* level of functioning are difficult to reconcile with the conceptual schemes that have proved their value on the ego and id level. Seen from the vantage point of the ego they actually appear as symptoms of irregularity in the orderly course of events—so much so that our current scientific system of thought is still inclined to disregard or explain away their very occurrence. There is an unmistakable similarity between this attitude and the one taken by the materialistic philosopher towards the appearance of purpose and meaning in human affairs: conflicting as it is with a rigid mechanistic scheme, it is conveniently kept outside his frame of reference and branded as the brain-child of the religious mystic or theologist philosopher.

Yet we have seen that under special circumstances certain patterns of stimulus and response can be observed which cannot satisfactorily be explained within our customary causal or teleological frame of reference. This does not, however, preclude their inclusion within a logically consistent conceptual scheme of its own. They can be classed under the heading of a *metalogical* series of events, providing a separate frame of reference for their proper appreciation.

Needless to say, however, the distinction between the three different conceptual schemes arrived at in this way is artificial. Teleological series are at the same time causally determined. Likewise, *psi* incidents are, as a general rule, part of the same teleological scheme which applies to the dynamics of mental processes in general. In particular we have seen that so-called tracer effects are capable of operational verification and therefore subject to the scientific method. In short, there are considerable areas of overlapping between the three conceptual schemes. Also, we must be aware of their intrinsic

<table>
<tr><th>Series</th><th>Mechanistic</th><th>Teleological</th><th>Metalogical</th></tr>
<tr><td>Guiding principle</td><td>Cause and effect</td><td>Purpose, final cause, "terminal focus"</td><td>Meaningful relationships</td></tr>
<tr><td>Basic philosophy</td><td>Newtonian mechanics, Darwinism</td><td>Thomistic theology, Free will</td><td>? ? ?</td></tr>
<tr><td rowspan="4">Practical application</td><td>Behaviourism, Pavlovian conditioning</td><td>Jurisprudence, Social science, Pedagogics</td><td>Parapsychology, ESP and PK experiments, Three-level therapy</td></tr>
<tr><td colspan="3">Psychosomatic Medicine</td></tr>
<tr><td colspan="3">Psychoanalysis (Freud, Adler, and Jung)</td></tr>
<tr><td colspan="3">Three-level therapy</td></tr>
<tr><td>Needed:</td><td colspan="3">A unified theory of science and psychology</td></tr>
</table>

TABLE 2.—Frames of reference.

Table 2 lists three different conceptual schemes which can be used for the understanding of world events. The mechanistic scheme is generally considered the one best suited for a strictly scientific approach. It can be contrasted with a teleological scheme which is traditionally applied to human affairs but is held to be incompatible with the scientific method. The third conceptual scheme conceives of world events in terms of a metalogical series, independent of the familiar laws of cause and effect but compatible with a revised and expanded system of psychodynamics based on the evaluation of meaningful relationships. The three conceptual schemes overlap in many areas suggesting the basic unity of world events which they seek to explain.

limitations. They do not carry us closer to anything like the ultimate scientific truth—even though the materialist philosopher, the teleologist, and the supernaturalist, each in his way, may solemnly affirm the sole and all-inclusive validity of his respective system of thought.

The mechanistic frame of reference is undoubtedly the most rewarding from the scientific point of view. It gives "all the answers" that arise in the fields of science and technology, including certain aspects of "human engineering." But it is inapplicable to many psychological problems—or at least the latter can more readily be treated by reference to goals and purposes postulated by the teleologist. The teleological scheme is thus superior to the mechanistic frame of reference whenever we are seeking a short cut towards the better understanding of human affairs. It serves as a convenient system of "abbreviations" in law, psychotherapy, and the social sciences, though its application to the rest of the world must remain a matter of personal preference.

Again, the metalogical frame of reference, while overlapping with the teleological scheme, is valid only within the limited range of scientifically verifiable *psi* occurrences. Beyond that it may easily amount to a throw-back to the fallacies of primitive magic or to the neurotic belief in the omnipotence of thought. It makes allowance for the extratemporal, extraspatial and a-causal aspects of the phenomena while at the same time the proper appreciation of their time- and space-structured, quantitative, aspects—or of their attending tracer effects—enables us to reconcile them with the mechanistic frame of reference used by the exact scientist.

Thus our proposed triad of conceptual schemes is capable of doing justice to the seemingly paradoxical, amphibious, nature of *psi* functions and in so doing paves the way for their systematic investigation and ultimate control in the psychotherapeutic situation—and in human affairs at large.

CHAPTER XX

Analytic Schools and Telepathic Leakage

IN the first two parts of the present study we have chiefly been concerned with specific telepathic incidents observed in the psychoanalytic situation, with their psychodynamic aspects and their broader implications upon personality structure and interpersonal relationships. Focusing attention on the psychological setting in both patient and therapist we found that in the majority of cases it is the therapist's unconscious conflicts or preconscious preoccupations with certain emotionally coloured wishes and expectations of his own which make their appearance in the patient's telepathic productions.

In many observations these preconscious preoccupations relate to the therapist's personal problems striking responsive chords in the patient's mind. But preoccupation with personal problems of this kind is by no means the only factor responsible for telepathy from the therapist to his patients. He may find to his surprise that some of their responses reflect his own emotionally charged interest in the subject-matter of telepathic communication itself.

This is suggested not only by highly specific tracer elements in the material concerned but also by the fact that the number of telepathic incidents encountered by the present writer—and by a few associates working along the same lines—is much larger than the number gathered by other therapists. It was also noted that the incidents occurred in smaller or larger droves or clusters, at periods of the therapist's heightened interest in and emotional preoccupation with his problem. Such observations were discussed in more detail in Chapters IV, V, and VI. They have likewise been described by Jule Eisenbud,[33e] Geraldine Pederson-Krag,[93, a] Montague Ullman,[133b] W. H. Gillespie,[52a] and others.

Observations like these suggest that more generally speaking, a favourable psychological setting may not be conducive to a few isolated telepathic incidents only but may create a more or less sustained telepathic susceptibility to highly complex motivational systems prevailing in the mind of a potential agent. They also tend to confirm the rule that the lesser an agent's conscious awareness of his own emotionally charged motivations the greater is their potential telepathic activity. It is this unintentional effect of preconscious motivations and attitudes which is here described as telepathic leakage and it is precisely the unintentional, preconscious nature of such leakage which makes it a matter of prime importance in the present context. As long as the therapist remains unaware of its operation telepathic leakage may easily influence the result of his analytic inquiry and thus become a potential source of error vitiating his conclusions. But it is readily understood that telepathic leakage may also play an important part outside the field proper of psychotherapy. Experimental psychology, by paying more attention to what can be described as para-experimental telepathy, might find an unexpected explanation of some of its conflicting or seemingly paradoxical findings.

How, then, are the therapist's unconscious attitudes, wishes and expectations capable of affecting his clinical observations and his scientific theorizing? The question, when applied to our contemporary schools of psychotherapy, is apt to raise so many controversial issues that it may be well to begin by throwing a brief glance upon systems of thought historically and culturally sufficiently removed from our own to permit their dispassionate discussion.

Mesmer's spectacular results with his *baquet* filled with magnetized iron filings may serve as our first example. His patients produced all the manifestations he expected them to produce including, sometimes, an improvement in their conditions. (That he probably obtained additional effects closely related to *psi* is another matter.) Hysteriform fits induced may have facilitated release of emotional tension in his patients and probably brought about similar phenomena in others by contagion. All this can easily be brushed aside today as the effect of mass hypnosis or mass hysteria. For Mesmer, however, his patients' reactions seemed to confirm his theories of animal magnetism and mysterious stellar influences upon humans in both health and disease.

The surgeon Dr. Braid, of Manchester, following the lead of Mesmer and his disciples, has been the first medical practitioner to recognize the hypnotic nature of these phenomena. But he, too, was led astray by some of the pseudo-scientific theories current in his time. His patients seemed to confirm all the bizarre beliefs held by the phrenologists concerning diverse mental faculties thought to be localized in various parts of the brain. Dr. Gardner Murphy[86b] quotes Braid's report about a woman who, while in the Mesmeric trance, gave ample demonstration of these wonders. "Under adhesiveness and friendship she clasped me, and on stimulating the organ of combativeness on the opposite side of the head, with the arm of that side, she struck two gentlemen (who she imagined were about to attack me) in such a manner as nearly laying one on the floor whilst with the other arm she held me in the most friendly manner. Under benevolence she seemed quite overwhelmed with compassion"—and so on and so forth.

Now we know full well that the ideas of the phrenologists were no less mistaken than Mesmer's theories of animal magnetism. But we have no reason to doubt the genuineness of Braid's observations. They suggest that, apart from the possible effects of unconscious conditioning or imitation, they were due to telepathic leakage resulting in apparent corroboration of the experimenter's pet scientific ideas.

The question as to whether or not telepathic leakage was involved in the spectacular clinical demonstrations of Charcot's *grande hysterie* in the Salpetrière in Paris is more difficult to decide. The gradual disappearance of cases of this type since the turn of the century is a matter of historic record. It may well be assumed that much of the symptomatology of what Charcot and his associates described as the hysteric *arc de circle*, as the *attitudes passionelles*, as well as the various stages of hypnotic trance studied by the Nancy school of hypnotism were artifacts and largely the result of unconscious conditioning by the operator.

Yet we also know that hypnosis itself is a condition eminently suitable for the emergence of telepathic phenomena. In fact the first observations of this kind were made in "mesmerized" subjects. In 1887 the French physician Dr. Azam[6] made experiments with telepathic "transmission" of tastes upon hypnotized persons. Pierre Janet and Dr. Gilbert[62] carried out a series of experiments with the celebrated subject Leonie involving hypnosis "at a distance." They claim that sixteen out of twenty-two tests of this kind have been successful. There is a vast number of more recent experiments which tend to confirm the role of hypnotism as a predisposing factor of telepathic phenomena. They are described in the relevant literature and need not be discussed here in greater detail.

But there are two modern instances of hypnotism or waking suggestion used for clinical and experimental purposes which call for comment. In one case overt hypnosis is applied to induce the subject to project himself into his childhood years in order to re-live and re-enact forgotten traumatic experiences and to retrieve repressed memories. This is the method of age regression introduced by Erickson and Kubie,[35] Wolberg[137] and their associates. Our second example is based on the pseudo-scientific exploitation of the method of age regression, known by the name of dianetics.[57] In both instances there is reason to suspect that occasionally undetected telepathic leakage from the hypnotist to his subject may be involved in the observations reported in the literature.

The case of a male homosexual published by F. I Regardie[98] in the *Psychiatric Quarterly* illustrates this point. The treatment consisted of hypnoanalysis based on hypnotically induced dreams, making ample use of the method of age regression. During forty sessions, S. P., a married man of thirty-eight, produced a remarkable series of dreams which Dr. Regardie describes as "unparalleled" in his twelve years' experience as a therapist. Never before had he encountered "dreams so dramatic, eloquent in their revelation or precise in their dynamic implications." He soon discovered that S. P. was "an ideal hypnotic patient" and could be "made to dream of any topic, about any conflict or any person in his background—

dreams that were far more dynamic, direct and clear than any nocturnal dream."

In effect, castration dreams, Oedipal dreams, dreams highlighting the struggle between instinctual drives and the superego could be produced to order. In the first hypnotic session described by Dr. Regardie the patient was made to regress to the age of six and recalled the following experience: "Mother likes daddy very much. She is always very nice to him and so glad when he comes home. . . . I know mummy needs daddy so I don't wish daddy to go away too badly. I felt bad in wishing daddy to go away." In one of the next sessions he can see a "large figure dominating everything. She is mother and looks like a Madonna. She is tall and big and at her feet is a child tugging and pulling at her skirt" and he goes on to say "She was all I needed for quite a long time, satisfying all my sexual needs. . . . Girls interested me mainly because they were small replicas of mother and therefore substituting for her. . . . Could not have sexual escapades with them because I could not have them with mother. . . . I must never have intercourse with any woman because that would in turn destroy mother. Homosexuality and masturbation were the only alternatives," etc.

Here, again, as in the case of Dr. Braid, there is no reason to doubt the genuineness of the observations described nor the veracity of Dr. Regardie's account. Moreover, his dynamic interpretations of the patient's productions are on much safer grounds than Braid's gratuitous phrenological concepts. Yet any experienced analyst will share Dr. Regardie's own wonderment at the facility with which the patient answered his prayers for a dynamic elucidation of Mr. S. P.'s conflict. How could such deeply repressed unconscious content as was obtained from the patient be mobilized right in the initial stages of the treatment? How are we to account for its perfect —nearly too perfect—agreement with current psychoanalytical tenets?

Certainly, it may simply be taken as an added confirmation of the validity of our theories. But have not the magnetopaths, phrenologists or spiritualists of a past era been equally gratified with spurious observations amounting to apparent confirmation of their beliefs? The question is: in cases like those described by Dr. Regardie how can telepathic leakage be excluded? Or, put in other words: in what way, if any, can telepathically induced attitudes, reflecting the hypnotist's own emotionally coloured wishes and expectations, be separated from what can rightly be regarded as the patient's own, autopsychic productions?

The method of dianetics leads us far off the field of scientifically oriented psychiatry to a sector occupied by cultist and sectarian practices surviving on the fringes of our contemporary civilization. Inaugurated by L. R. Hubbard,[57] originally known as an imaginative science fiction writer, dianetics seems to owe part of its success to the extravagant claims of curing virtually all diseases, organic or functional, ranging from cancer to claustrophobia. Not less striking is the claim of the dianetician to carry his subject back on the "time track" to his early infantile or even pre-natal experiences. Thus an auditor, i.e. a practitioner of dianetics, in all seriousness, related the following story to the present writer: Six subjects or *preclears* were carried back on the time track to their pre-natal, pre-embryonal lives. They were made to recall the engrams or memory traces pertaining to their existence as spermatozoa, prior to fertilization of the maternal egg. None of the subjects, the auditor asserted, had any knowledge of the biological process of fertilization. Yet they described in great detail the course taken by the sperm, the histological structure of the spermatozoa themselves, the ciliary movements of their tails, and so on and so forth.

It would be easy to discard fanciful accounts of this kind as nothing but a gigantic and well-advertised hoax. But their importance lies in the fact that they spur the imagination of thousands of credulous people and thus may pave the way for occasional therapeutically effective suggestions which an equally ignorant if self-assured operator may throw in into the bargain. Obviously, cures effected by such a method are to be explained much in the same way as those achieved by the primitive medicine man, the quack or charlatan by purely magical procedures. So far as apparent confirmation of theoretical concepts is concerned here, too, as in the case of

Mesmer's animal magnetism, or Braid's phrenomagnetism, telepathic leakage may account for that part of the observations which is not due to mere misrepresentations by the therapist or cryptomnesia on the part of the subject.

But it would be unfair to brush aside all claims coming from dianetic quarters as mere figments of imagination. Their material may well contain a grain of truth. One part may be of the same order as that afforded by serious clinical studies applying the method of age regression. Another part may be due to telepathic leakage from the operator to his subject. Similar considerations apply to countless other methods of faith-healing which have reached brief periods of fame—or notoriety—in the past decades.

How, then, does our insight into the part played by telepathic leakage in primitive, pre-scientific systems of psychotherapy help towards its recognition and utilization in our approach? First and foremost, we have to be aware of telepathy as a possible source of error leading to spurious confirmation of our own scientific theories. The first step towards this end is to include the therapist's counter-transference in a systematic way within the frame of reference of the treatment. This is meant by the method of comparative analysis of both the therapist and the patient. Secondly, we have to re-examine a substantial part of the evidence afforded by the various schools of psychoanalysis from our point of view. It goes without saying that this is not the place or the time to undertake such a formidable task. But it is high time for us to realize that it is not necessarily the poorly-trained therapist who is subject to the fallacies that are apt to arise from telepathic leakage. It may well be that it is just his previous training and analytic indoctrination which has so imbued him with a ready-made set of ideas and scientific expectations as to make him quite unaware of their presence in his mental make-up.

Some of the mutually contradictory—yet nevertheless perfectly plausible—findings arrived at by the rival schools may thus find a satisfactory explanation: their divergencies are due to different theoretical premises and presuppositions held by their protagonists and, as a result of telepathic leakage, are faithfully reflected by their patients.

To avoid confusion which may easily arise from this state of affairs we have to distinguish between three principal aspects of the material with which we are confronted in the psychoanalytic situation: (1) superficial, culturally determined content; (2) content determined by the impact of the therapist's personality—and by his personal bias—upon his patients; and (3) content pertaining exclusively to the patient's personality, to his autopsychic sphere—provided that such content can altogether be isolated in pure culture.

A simple example may illustrate the point. If a patient treated by a Freudian or Adlerian or Jungian analyst dreams that his motor-car has been stolen the manifest content of his dream is obviously culturally determined. Again, the interpretation of such a dream in terms of castration fears, inferiority feelings, or the like, is largely a matter of the individual therapist's personal bias. In the last analysis general agreement as to the "real" meaning of such a dream is perhaps impossible to reach.

True telepathic leakage goes, however, beyond cultural conditioning. For instance, Jung's patients, at certain periods of his work, seemed to furnish ample evidence of uncommon abilities and hyperfunctions of the unconscious. Sometimes they contained grandiose allusions to ancient Egyptian or Assyrian or Hindu texts. At other times they seemed to bear out some of the fanciful beliefs of medieval astrologers and alchemists. No Freudian or Adlerian analyst seems to have ever recorded material of this kind. Yet I, for myself, have noticed peculiar changes in the dream imagery used by my patients at various periods of my analytic work. The changes seemed to be largely conditioned by my own preoccupation with the dream material encountered in the records of various analytic schools. The frankly telepathic repercussions of my later preoccupation with the problem of telepathy are amply demonstrated by the material described in the first part of this book.

One could object at this point that all these discrepancies simply reflect changes within the general outlook of both patient and therapist, reinforced by their community of interests and intellectual preoccupations. This is a perfectly legitimate objection—but it only holds true for cases in which the transmission of specific material from the therapist to the patient can be explained in terms of overt verbal communication. It is not applicable to such observations as form the main topic of the present study. They are at bottom all due to telepathic leakage, that is they are findings whose dismissal as being merely due to telepathic leakage would only amount to an added confirmation of our thesis.

But I have already pointed out elsewhere[32] that whatever be the extent of telepathic leakage in the making of our theories, there is ample evidence available which precludes telepathic falsification of the material upon which our conclusions are based. Such evidence is supplied by biographical material, diaries, works of art, and other recorded data which can be subjected to systematic analysis. It is further supported by psychoanalytic appraisal of anthropological observations derived from other cultures such as was first attempted in Freud's celebrated *Totem and Taboo*. Data obtained from such objective sources serve as collateral evidence in support of conclusions arrived at in the psychoanalytic situation.

Another argument in their favour derives from the empirical fact that the unconscious is not readily accessible to outside influences. It may be affected by the emotional impact of the analytic situation as a whole; it may be moved like the sea lashed by a storm—or rippled by a breeze—but its basic composition is not likely to be changed. Its surface may be contaminated by an oil film left by the oceanographers' vessel passing by, but the chances are that a sample lifted from below comes very close to the real thing.

We have to realize, furthermore, that even though some of the material produced by the patient may be due to telepathic leakage, that is, derived from the therapist's unconscious rather than from that of the patient, the strict distinction which is usually made between the two no longer applies to the level on which telepathic leakage comes about. The occurrence of telepathic leakage may affect some of the conclusions drawn from the individual case but does not invalidate Freud's basic dynamic and genetic propositions.

This should be borne in mind on seeking to evaluate the

criticisms levelled against one another by the protagonists of rival schools. To quote just one example of controversy: the objections raised by Edward Glover[50] as to the universal nature of Jung's archetypes is certainly justified. The concept of the Golden Age, of the Eternal Feminine or of the Virgin Birth cannot possibly be considered as revelations of an ultimate psychic truth. Such ideas, unless they have been intellectualized and put through the process of anapsychic organization, cannot be assimilated by our thinking. This is why they bear the imprint of Jung's personality and of the culture in which he has been reared. But we should not forget that precisely the same is true for Freud's castration complex or Oedipus complex, or for such minor additions to the psychoanalytic vocabulary as the Electra or Bruenhilde complex; for Rank's[97a] primal conflict or for what in Chapter XVI of this book has been described as the conflict of psychomitosis. In short, we have to realize that at bottom all our insight into psychic reality is subject to telepathic leakage or is otherwise culturally determined. It is therefore valid only within a limited frame of reference.

This state of affairs is not, however, confined to the domain of psychology and psychoanalysis. Goethe's famous saying: "Alles Vergaengliche ist nur ein Gleichnis"* is equally true for the psychic universe of Freud as for the physical world of Einstein. Still, the Einstein equations, however remote from the ultimate physical reality they may be, serve as convenient tools for our grappling with the physical world on the ego level. In the same way Freud's topographic, economic, and genetic formulations well serve their purpose within their frame of reference and are likely to do so for many years to come.

It is true that paying proper attention to the telepathic factor involved in interpersonal relationships is undoubtedly apt to modify the original Freudian doctrine. Some of the adjustments that may become necessary have already been indicated in the chapters dealing with the ego, the id, and *psi* and with personality structure in general. But it will be noted that such basic operational concepts as repression, projection,

* All things mortal are but a simile.

identification, displacement, etc., have been adopted here without the need for major modifications. Indeed, without them some of the conclusions presented here would have been impossible to reach. Again, so far as analytic interpretations are concerned, our newly gained insight does not detract from their pragmatic validity—provided that due attention is paid to the part played by telepathic leakage in their formulation. We have to realize that psychoanalytic interpretations, far from being the fruits of the analyst's superior knowledge or intelligence, are the results of his joint experience with the patient—of an experience in which partial insight gained by one may spark the achievement of more insight by the other.

One is again reminded at this point of the way in which progress has been made in the physical sciences. When the Russian chemist Mendeleyev evolved his periodic system of elements some sixty years ago, a basic feat of scientific discovery was accomplished. Some of the crude atomic concepts upon which his system had been based have now been abandoned and replaced by more up-to-date knowledge concerning the micro-structure of the atom. Nevertheless, one atom of oxygen still combines with two atoms of hydrogen and will presumably continue to do so even when some of the recent formulations of nuclear physics have yielded to a still newer theory of atomic structure. Much in the same way, whatever new discoveries regarding personality structure and psychodynamics can be expected in the future, they are unlikely to affect the principal findings of modern dynamic psychiatry made by Freud, Adler, Jung, and their followers.

There is only one basic difference between the physicist's and the psychologist's approach which must not be overlooked. Barring the controversial effects of psychokinesis, the behaviour of atoms or protons or electrons is unlikely to be influenced by the mental attitudes of those engaged in their investigation.*

* The German physicist Pascual Jordan has pointed out that such a statement is in need of qualification when applied to the field of modern quantum mechanics. Even when studying the behaviour of an electron "we cannot make observations without changing at the same time the state of the object." ("Reflections on Parapsychology, Psychoanalysis, and Atomic Physics," *J. Parapsychol.*, 15, 1951.)

Yet we have seen that in the study of interpersonal relationships telepathic leakage from the observer to the subject may well be capable of having just such an effect. No psychological theory that fails to make allowance for this fact can feel quite sure of its ground and no school of psychotherapy can claim to be truly scientific unless it is aware of the part played by this factor.

CHAPTER XXI

How Does the Patient Respond?

IF our discussion of the problem presented by telepathic leakage gave the impression that telepathy in the psychoanalytic situation is nothing but an embarrassment to psychoanalytic practice and theory such an impression has to be corrected. Whatever challenge for a revision and restatement of individual findings it may imply, it also opens up new therapeutic possibilities. Clearly, telepathic leakage need not be confined to the transmission of cognitive or ideational content. It may also embrace motivations and inner attitudes of the therapist more intimately related to the ultimate purpose of the treatment.

What, then, are the therapeutic potentialities of the telepathic factor involved in the doctor-patient relationship? Before we are ready to go into the merits of this question we must make one more brief digression. We have to review the case histories of our patients from a new angle and seek to evaluate the nature of their responses to the telepathic incidents which have come to our notice.

In doing so we have to realize two things. First, it is not altogether permissible to take a given telepathic incident out of its context and regard it as an isolated "incident." Secondly, we must not forget that the response to such a purportedly isolated incident, like the response to experiences of all denominations, both autopsychic and heteropsychic, need not necessarily be direct, immediate or obvious. Like the patient's reactions to many and varied life situations it may be subdued and barely perceptible; it may be repressed or shifted to other areas; it may be confined to symbolically disguised or distorted reaction patterns; or it may manifest itself in reaction formations and such tendencies of denial or isolation as are familiar in the picture of compulsion neurosis. It may call forth an attitude of detachment bordering on depersonalization, or even provoke such forms of negativistic or frankly catatonic behaviour as can be seen in full-fledged schizophrenics.

It is perhaps these many and varied types of reactions to telepathy which offer an added explanation for the comparative rarity of unmistakably telepathic occurrences observed in daily life. Only a few bottles containing a telepathic "message" are properly sealed, labelled, and addressed before they are thrown into the sea. Only in the few instances discussed in the preceding chapters has the therapist—and some of his patients—become aware of the incidents. Many more "bottles" have sunk to the bottom of the sea. Even so, in the majority of cases, the incident observed blended imperceptibly with the ordinary run of the patient's life. But for the fact of his undergoing analytic treatment with the present writer it would perhaps never have come to light.

Ruth, the first patient, whose case was described in Chapter III, remained unaware of the telepathic nature of her dream featuring the therapist's apartment. The same is true for the dream of Ronald H. derived in part from my unsuccessful search for a summer house. In both cases there was nothing in the patient's attitude to betray the heteropsychic derivation of the material concerned. Their reaction was confined to the assimilation of the telepathic element and its integration with the rest of their waking experience, especially with the dynamics of the existing transference relationship.

This is also well illustrated by the following dream dreamt in the second week of analysis by Mr. H., a patient of fifty-three. "I walked along a canal; it was quite straight and there were dams on both sides. It resembled a lake. Along with me walked two women and a boy, about five years old. Then I tried to phone somebody, I don't know whom, but the connection was cut. But then I found the wires, put them together and could establish the connection. Then I walked around a square several city blocks large. I thought I saw something like the Eiffel Tower and the Champs Élysées at a distance. The earth of the dam was like freshly ploughed earth, but not like arable land. It was like sea dunes or sand in the desert and the whole terrain went up and down and up and down." He illustrated the formation of the terrain by drawing a sinusoidal curve.

The dreamer's associations in connection with the dream led him back to his childhood years and reminded him of walks he took with his family. The little boy was the dreamer himself. The telephone wires reminded him of calling his mother. The hilly ground brought back memories of a picture book he liked to look at as a little boy, and so on and so forth.

The striking fact is that here, again, the manifest content

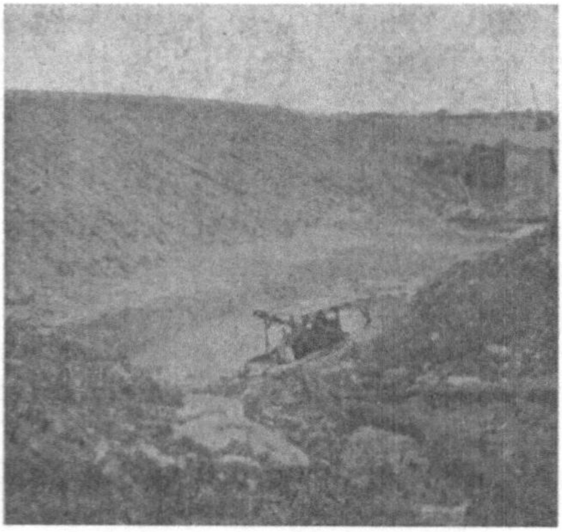

FIG. 12.—The therapist's Sunday walk.

of the dream contained elements which showed close correspondence with trivial incidents on my side of the picture at the time the dream occurred. As it happened, on the Sunday morning preceding the dream I had taken a walk with my wife and my daughter in our neighbourhood. We wanted to have a close look at what we used to call our private Champs Élysées, that is, an area of wooded wasteland off the outlying parts of Queens Boulevard through which a new connecting highway to Idlewild Airport was to be built. Huge mounds of earth cut through the hilly terrain as shown in the picture above. Looking down to the levelled ground in which rainwater had accumulated indeed gave the impression of a dam being built. The mounds of earth dug up by the bulldozers had a sandy colour. Proceeding from our "dam," we continued on our walk by skirting the adjacent Maplegrove Cemetery which occupies several city blocks and returned home. Charting our walk on a street map would amount to a rectangle of about a mile square. I may also mention the structure of a big water tower which dominated the view from the far side of the "dam."

In order to verify, if possible, the telepathic nature of the dream I took a photograph of the "dam" to which we paid a visit on our Sunday walk and showed it to Mr. H., together with nine more photos featuring such diverse objects as a building in a park, a group of people in front of a farm-house, etc. The patient was asked to tell me if any of the pictures reminded him of one of his recent dreams. Mr. H. pointed without hesitation to the photograph of the "dam," though without the show of any sign of actual recognition or surprise.

It is interesting to note that the *motif* of the broken and restored communication, symbolized by the wires in the manifest content of the dream, seemed to contain a direct reference to telepathy between the therapist and the patient, with the former playing the part of the mother with whom Mr. H. was anxious to establish and maintain contact.* Indeed, no other explanation can account for the surrealistic inclusion of this element in the manifest content of the dream.

As indicated, however, the patient had been utterly unaware of the telepathic implications of his dream and remained so even after the inquiry into his reaction to the photographs. The same is true for Mrs. M., whose telepathic dreams featuring a social gathering in the present writer's home were described in Chapter XVII. In both cases the whole context in which the dreams occurred did not warrant the disclosure of their telepathic implications to the dreamer.

Sometimes, however, the dreamer may become aware with dramatic force of the unusual nature of his experience. I may only recall my own dream described in Chapter VII to emphasize the violent emotional impact which may be attached to an

* Eisenbud[33e] has specifically called attention to the fact that telephones and other means of long-distance communication are often used as symbols of telepathic communication in the manifest content of the dream.

occasional telepathic element breaking into the autopsychic sphere. In the dream I found myself exposed to the humiliating situation which on analysis could be connected with an angry outburst of my patient Ronald H. accusing me of a professionally unbecoming attitude. In this instance the dreamer's response to the heteropsychic material was immediately apparent although its offensive connotation was shifted to the infantile level and, to soften the blow, the accuser was put on a plane with Nazi fanatics whose case had sufficiently been discredited since the downfall of Germany. It will also be noted that part of the sting had been taken out of Ronald's invective by the simple device of silencing his verbal outburst against me and making him pass the Nazi newspaper to the dreamer without a word of comment.

A classical example of displacement and distortion brought to bear upon telepathic material is illustrated by Freud's first observation[44] relating to a presumptively telepathic dream. In this case the father of a married daughter dreamt that his second wife had given birth to twins. As it happened, it was his daughter from his first marriage who had been delivered of twins on the same night, about one month earlier than her confinement was expected.

Freud suggests in his analysis of the dream that it may express the dreamer's unconscious wish to be father to his daughter's child. Yet since such an incestuous wish is intolerable to his conscience it is displaced from his daughter to his wife, thus disguising his unconscious incestuous desire. It is readily understood that failing such elaborate displacement and disguise the telepathic material concerned may have altogether been barred from his consciousness.

In an earlier observation of my own[32] a young woman had a telepathic dream featuring the death of the wife of an elderly friend whom she held in high regard. The woman's death had actually occurred on the night of the dream and the dream itself satisfied an unconscious wish of the dreamer to take her mother's place by the side of a beloved father figure. Yet except for the anxiety felt in the dream nothing betrayed its hidden Oedipal significance. This, in turn, made it possible for the dreamer herself to recognize its telepathic nature.

A more recent observation illustrates the same principle. It is at the same time a graphic example of telepathy between mother and daughter, reminiscent of the so-called Phantasms of the Dying, described by the early workers in psychical research. Lottie is now a woman of forty, a native of Prague. She and her husband came to this country in 1938. Owing to circumstances beyond her control she was forced to leave her widowed mother, aged fifty-three, behind in a country threatened by the Nazis. Lottie was torn with remorse for having done so and she continued to do all in her power to obtain a visa for the elderly lady and to bring her over to the U.S.A. On April 12, 1939, between 10 and 10.30 a.m., Lottie was suddenly overcome by a feeling of anxiety and restlessness. She had a sense of some impending disaster and went into an uncontrollable crying fit. This happened in her apartment in New York. Helen, her maid, tried her best to calm her down and to find out the reason for Lottie's anxiety. But all Lottie could tell her was that she felt something terrible had happened to her mother—or maybe to her mother-in-law. Helen's consolation that she would not have to cry so bitterly if something had happened to her mother-in-law did not help matters. Lottie rushed to the phone and tried to put through a transatlantic telephone call to her mother. Owing to technical difficulties this was not possible. She shared her anxiety with her husband and on the next morning went to her safe deposit vault to parcel out what family heirlooms she had brought from the old country so that her mother, on her arrival here, would have an equal share of the jewels—provided she would ever arrive. On her return from the bank Lottie's husband broke to her the news that on the night from April 12th to 13th her mother had suddenly passed away. The cable, sent by a relative, mentioned a carbuncle for which she had an operation. But Lottie learned a month later that her mother's death had been a suicide. On the critical night she had opened the gas jets in her apartment. Making allowance for the six hours' time difference between Prague and New York Lottie's anxiety attack may have occurred after a latency period of several hours following her mother's mortal crisis. As in many cases of this kind there is, however, no information available as to the exact time she had succumbed to the gas poisoning.

Lottie's case is wholly in the tradition of the older reports found in the literature of psychical research. But in this instance psychoanalytic inquiry helped to throw more light upon its dynamics. Lottie's behaviour shows that the telepathic "message" provoked three different reactions in the percipient: (1) she tried to attach her anxiety to the fate of her mother-in-law; that is, she displaced the telepathic impression gained to another person; (2) she sought to deny its reality by the symbolic gesture of parcelling out her jewellery as though her mother was still alive; (3) in so doing she allayed her guilt feelings which were connected with her mother's death. In short, in this case, the telepathic impression was subjected to the well-known mechanisms of displacement, denial, and reaction formation.

Whether or not heteropsychic material finds its way into the autopsychic sphere without being stripped of all attending identification marks that might facilitate its detection depends on the general conditions in which the incident occurs. Some of the telepathic episodes described in the case of Fred L. provoked his openly negativistic reactions to the therapist. But for the previous undistorted incidents of the same kind their telepathic nature would have probably never been recognized. Again, in many cases telepathy remains undetected because sufficiently strong defensive mechanisms are at work in both agent and percipient to block its transition into the conscious sphere.

That *psi* may nevertheless play an important part even in schizophrenic patients was pointed out in some detail in my book *Telepathy and Medical Psychology*. Two conclusions drawn from the observations discussed there may be quoted here. First, the schizoid type of personality may show a striking lack of sensitivity to various social situations. He may be colour-blind, as it were, to the moods, feelings, and emotional attitudes of his fellow-men. Yet at the same time he may develop something like a selective telepathic sensitiveness to repressed hostility in his social environment of which his friends and relatives may themselves be unaware on the conscious level.

As a general rule the barriers preventing the breakthrough

of such material are sufficiently tight. Indeed it is the excessive tightness of these barriers which may account for part of the patient's insensitivity to his social environment. Again, in some schizoid individuals we find a paradoxical mixture of insensitiveness and hypersensitivity which may make their adjustment to the group still more precarious. Overly sensitive to the attitudes of his fellow-men, the patient may develop what Wilhelm Reich[100] described as the protective armour-plating of character. This armour-plating, while offering only a modicum of protection, may lead to an increasing isolation and detachment from his fellows resulting in the typical "withdrawn," "shut-in" type of personality. E. Kretschmer[71] described this aspect of the schizoid type of personality as his *psychesthetic proportion.*

The two alternating attitudes are well illustrated by the following observation. A woman of forty-one, a borderline schizophrenic, reported two dreams in two consecutive sessions. (1) "I am in a house and the house is surrounded by another layer of house. A storm is beating against it." This dream expresses clearly the neurotic defences the schizoid type of personality seeks to build up as an extra protection from dangers threatening from within and from without.

(2) "I am in a house which is in a state of breaking up. All my possessions are kept in open shelves; there are no closets or wardrobes. I try to pick up my possessions and salvage what I can lay hands on." This dream shows with equal clarity the threatening breakdown of ego defences—the uncanny "openness" of schizophrenic personality structure.

This does not, however, necessarily spell the impending doom of the patient. In a recent paper Montague Ullman[133a] has called attention to the fact that many borderline schizophrenics may maintain (or develop?) the capacity of using their heteropsychic sensitiveness for a constructive purpose. It may serve them as a means of compensatory communication with their fellow-men on the *psi* level, making up for their blocking on the ego level.

In advanced schizophrenics the picture is different. In these cases the breakdown of the barriers separating the ego from the non-ego may be complete and the non-ego itself assumes nothing but a hostile, menacing connotation to the patient. His failure to ward off the maddening influx of heteropsychic material—or to subject it at least to some measure of catapsychic breakdown and disorganization—may result in the psychological equivalent of an anaphylactic shock: the patient may lapse into a catatonic stupor. The state of regression reached by these patients has given rise to many interesting speculations about the nature of the schizophrenic process. Bleuler,[11] Jung,[65b] and especially Storch[123] described the peculiar archaic modes of thinking that make their appearance at this stage as developmental throwbacks, due to an unconscious recall or recapitulation of the early phylogenetic history of our race. Whether and how far, on the other hand, some of the bizarre visions of cosmic catastrophes described by such patients may with equal justification be taken as allusions to a vague foreknowledge of man's ultimate downfall at the conclusion of our much-heralded atomic age must, in the absence of tracer elements and of any means of verification, remain a matter of still more gratuitous speculation.

On rare occasions, however, an unmistakable tracer element may betray the struggle of the schizoid type of personality in warding off heteropsychic influences. Mr. O., aged twenty-nine, had been undergoing treatment for character neurosis. A gifted writer of science fiction, he was suffering from social anxiety, painfully aware of his own emotional blocking and flatness of affect. At the same time he had marked difficulties in mastering his excessive sensitiveness in all social situations. One day my secretary asked him on my behalf to change his usual Tuesday appointment from 5 p.m. to 6 p.m. He agreed and my secretary made the necessary adjustment in her diary. Yet I, for my part, had failed to do so in my desk calendar and still expected him at 5 p.m. Mr. O. appeared right on time—i.e. on the wrong time scheduled in my calendar. He emphatically disclaimed any recollection of my secretary's telephone call in which she had asked him for the change two days ago. When we agreed to proceed with the session despite my other commitments he remarked that while on the way to my office he had "known" beforehand something would go wrong with our appointment. He was reproachful and hostile and felt rejected by the therapist. In fact, he remained so for the ensuing two to three weeks of his analysis.

Certainly, this attitude could be attributed to the break of routine forced on the patient by the suggested change of schedule. He had, however, readily consented to such changes on past occasions and had no apparent reason for refusing to co-operate this time. He was in no way inconvenienced by a one-hour postponement of his session, nor was there anything in what transpired during the subsequent hours to account for his unusual irritability and resentment. There was only one factor which had been added this time to the total situation: my forgetting the postponement of his appointment. Whatever was the reason for my forgetfulness, the fact is that I expected him at 5 p.m. instead of at 6 p.m., while we have to assume that the patient still felt duty bound, as it were, to appear at 5 p.m. instead of at 6 p.m.

It is not easy to unravel the complex dynamics of this situation. Yet viewed from the angle of the telepathy hypothesis the patient's behaviour is readily understood. His previous telephone conversation with my secretary on the one hand and my own confusion as to the exact time of his appointment on the other put him under two contradictory orders to which he responded like one of Pavlov's experimental animals exposed to two conflicting stimuli: he stalled, became anxious, irritable and hostile.

It should be noted at this point that the patient, despite his unmistakable resistance to heteropsychic influences, as well as to any and every close personal contact with his fellows in general, had on repeated previous occasions shown evidence of telepathic susceptibility. Indeed it may well be assumed that it was precisely his need to forestall the repetition of incidents of the kind described above which caused him to withdraw into his shell, to become the reserved, introvert, shut-in type of personality as which he made his way through life.

It is interesting to contrast this reaction with a similar incident which occurred during the winding up period of Ronald's H.'s treatment, whose case was described in Chapters IV and VII. This time a last-minute change in my schedule made a shift of his appointment from 5 p.m. to 1 p.m.

necessary. When told by my secretary that it would be impossible for me to reach him over the phone I reconciled myself to the inevitable, wondering how I would adjust my afternoon programme to Ronald's scheduled appointment. All the greater was my surprise when at 1 p.m. Ronald unexpectedly appeared in my office. He said he was not sure about the exact time our session was to take place: at 1 p.m. or 5 p.m. He had nothing else to do now so he thought he might just as well drop in and find out.

It is interesting to note that the patient's slip occurred at a period of pronounced positive transference which coincided with his marked progress in the resolution of his neurotic conflict. At about the same time two or three more telepathic incidents were recorded in his case history. I may also add that although Ronald was suffering from a compulsion neurosis which caused a certain rigidity in his character structure he was nevertheless of a typically extrovert personality type and in this respect the exact counterpart of the previous patient.

The implications of the two contrasting attitudes reflected by the two incidents described here are far-reaching enough. They indicate that potential telepathic influences emanating from the therapist may have two diametrically opposite effects. Telepathy may readily be adopted and assimilated by one type of personality, enhancing his positive transference. Alternatively, it may be resolutely rejected and warded off by another personality type and result in further increase of his original resistance to the treatment relationship.

Several examples of the two opposing reaction types have already emerged from our description. Ruth, the dreamer of the first dream discussed in this book, responded to the telepathic element involved with an attitude of sharing and identification. Her dream expressed her desire to be admitted to the therapist's family circle and to move with him into his new apartment. Telepathy, we said, was not only the result of but also the vehicle of positive transference in her case.

The same principle is illustrated by Mr. H.'s dream in which the patient literally joined the therapist on a Sunday walk with his wife and daughter. In this case the telepathic element contained in the dream was in effect the first indication of the patient's positive transference on a father figure. In the same vein, most of the telepathic incidents seen in the two friends Ronald and Fred, described in the first part of this book, were largely symptomatic of their positive transference on the therapist. Only one or two reactions of Fred L. were exceptions to this rule. But it should be noted that the personality make-up of this patient showed marked schizoid features and that his positive transference was on repeated occasions vitiated by periods of hostile withdrawal. Again, it should be recalled that Mr. T.'s apparently precognitive dream, described in Chapters VIII and IX, occurred at a time when the dreamer, an anxiety hysteric, had just succeeded in breaking down his initial resistance to the therapist and had become ready to accept him as a friend and helper. At the same time here, again, the dream coincided with a dramatic improvement of the patient's condition.

The contrast between the positive reaction type seen in the majority of patients reviewed here and the resistance and sense of frustration shown by the schizoid patient described above is unmistakable. It would become still more convincing if we were in a position to illustrate the negative reaction type by more instances tagged with clearly identifiable tracer elements. Yet it is needless to say that such cases cannot but be rare. For obvious reasons patients of this type are only too likely to succeed in repressing or warding off heteropsychic experiences of all denominations. Consequently there may be nothing left in their productions to tell the tale of their abortive telepathic susceptibility.

I hinted that personalities belonging to this group show a well-defined character structure. Their withdrawn, detached attitude is often associated with a striking lack of intuitive understanding of their fellows. They are unable to establish anything like a direct empathic or enkinetic response to them. Their basically defensive attitude blocks their tendency to put themselves into another person's "psychological shoes" and they are at a loss to understand how it feels to be in them. Their formal intelligence may be adequate or even high above average but they invariably fail to understand what makes another person "tick." They are apt to misunderstand his motivations and usually fail to convey a true picture of their own thoughts and motivations to others. Though they may possess considerable verbal dexterity an essential factor in their ability to communicate with their fellow-men is missing. To the sensory aphasic words have no meaning while the motor aphasic is incapable of expressing them through the medium of language. The personality type described here behaves like an aphasic in relation to *psi* both as far as understanding of and the conveyance of meaning on the *psi* level are concerned. If the term were not already used in a different connotation he could be described as *a-pathic*. He is suffering, neurologically speaking, from *empathic agnosia*.

There is, however, nothing to indicate a constitutional origin of the "a-pathic" personality type. All the available evidence rather indicates that it has to be regarded as a special reaction type due to early infantile difficulties of communication with parental figures. That it is precisely personalities habitually insensitive of or desensitized to *psi* who are also apt to develop schizophrenic psychoses is another matter.

On the opposite end of the personality scale we find persons who are endowed with particular "psychic" or intuitive proclivities. They possess, or claim to possess, unfailing hunches, a particular flair for judging people; they may state that they are able to "get" their personalities in a "flash." They are highly sensitive to people's moods, to the atmosphere in their social environment. More often than not this is associated with a keen power of observation, with an increased sensitiveness to sounds, smells or colours. By contrast to the peculiarities of the intuitively blocked or a-pathic reaction type, persons belonging to this category nowhere feel happier than in the group. They are sociable, outgoing, good mixers, and do well at jobs requiring leadership and social facility. It is interesting to note at this point that Cottrell and Dymond,[24] whose experimental studies on empathy were referred to in Chapter XII, have come to much the same conclusions in regard to persons reaching high scores in empathy. The reader familiar with Jung's[65c] typology will also note that Jung's extravert-intuitive type is in turn closely related to the personality of the so-called psychic or sensitive described in the literature of psychical research. That the latter reaction type may indeed be considered as a group of its own has been pointed out elsewhere.[32e] Yet here, again, we have to make the proviso that so-called psychic sensitiveness may be nothing but the result of habitual cultivation in persons whose original susceptibility to *psi*, instead of being stifled and suppressed, has persistently and methodically been encouraged. Alleged psychics may thus be the products of gradual cultural conditioning in an atmosphere of forbearance and social approbation.

What, then, is the relevance to our issue of the two contrasting reaction types discussed here? They are closely related to two contrasting reaction types which were discussed in some detail in earlier sections of this book. One is the relationship between parent and child; the other is the relationship between therapist and patient.

It will be recalled that our discussion of the child-parent relationship revealed two alternative types of reaction, closely reminiscent of those discussed here. We said that, on a deeper level, the child-parent relationship is governed by a tendency to vicarious functioning and empathic response. These two attitudes may be conducive either to a pattern of sharing, of ready acceptance and compliance with parental influences impinging upon the child, or else they may provoke a pattern of resistance, expressing the child's need for independence, his desire to sever the bonds tying him to his mother's personality. In extreme cases this struggle, unremitting and lifelong, may extend far beyond the physiological boundaries of parent and child. It may decisively influence the individual's attitude towards his elders, his superiors, and towards authority in general. We have also seen that the identical attitude of resistance may be duplicated in the psychoanalytic situation. It is closely connected with the patient's negative transference which, so long as it is unresolved, may offset, if not altogether nullify, the outcome of the treatment.

Alternatively, the patient may shift his original loyalty and affection from parental figures to the person of the analyst and establish a relationship of positive transference. As a general rule phases of positive transference alternate, however, with negative transference, or to put it in Freud's[44e] words, "transference is ambivalent, it comprises positive, affectionate as well as negative and hostile attitudes towards the analyst." And he adds: "The fact of transference is a factor of undreamt of importance—on the one hand an instrument of irreplaceable value and on the other a source of serious dangers." This is particularly true for that type of patient whose personality structure has developed in a constant struggle for survival in the face of excessive pressures from a possessive and demanding parent figure. Patients of this type may or may not be candidates for a potential schizophrenic breakdown. In any case, they are well-nigh incapable of developing what Freud described as a transference neurosis and have up to recently been considered unsuitable for the psychoanalytic approach.

The close dynamic and genetic relationship between early infantile conditioning and the two alternative patterns of transference brings two separate strands of our argument together again. If we are right in assuming that *psi* plays an important part in the growth and early development of the child we may be equally justified in expecting to find evidence of the same factor in the transference situation which, in the last analysis, is nothing else than a re-enactment of early infantile relationships on an adult level. Indeed, there are periods in the course of every analysis when the transference relationship is dominated by a marked tendency to regression to infantile patterns of behaviour. This may entail the development of psychosomatic and conversion symptoms hitherto absent in the clinical picture. But it may also enhance the patient's tendency to empathic sharing and compliance and make him eminently susceptible to heteropsychic influences of all kinds—including therapeutic suggestions—emanating from the analyst and communicated to him on the *psi* level.

The fact is that in the majority of observations reviewed here the actual telepathic incident occurred at periods of marked positive transference whereas hardly more than one or two incidents have come to our notice under conditions of negative transference. It is this direct, positive correlation between positive transference and telepathy which seems to justify our statement that telepathy may be both the result of and the vehicle for positive transference.

CHAPTER XXII

Telepathy: Cause or Effect?

OUR description of the two principal reaction types to telepathy which can be discerned in the psychoanalytic situation has gone far to show the close correlation between telepathy and psychoanalytic transference. A positive transference relationship seems to promote the occurrence of telepathy between therapist and patient. This point has originally been made by Freud[44] and was later specifically stressed by Servadio.[112] On the other hand telepathy may play the part of the Trojan horse, helping to smuggle the contraband of the therapist's counter-transference into the mind of the patient. In view of the all-important role of positive transference in psychotherapy this might easily lead to the conclusion that telepathy may indeed be a powerful factor in the dynamics of psychological treatment, psychoanalytic or otherwise. But is such a conclusion really justified? A condensed survey of the clinical observations discussed in this study shows that so long as we focus our attention on time- and space-structured tracer elements only such an inference is not borne out by the facts.

Table 3 features the eight patients in whom one or more unequivocal telepathic incidents have been observed in the

TABLE 3

Nr.	Patient	Diagnosis	Ref.: Chapter	Telepathy	Therapeutic Response
1.	Ruth	hysteria	III	++	+
2.	Ronald H.	compul. neur.	IV and VII	++	+
3.	Fred L.	compul. neur.	V, VI, and XXI	++	+
4.	Mr. T.	anx. hyster.	VIII and IX	+	+
5.	Mr. Z.	obsess. comp.	VII and IX	+	+
6.	Mrs. M.	neur. depres.	XVII	++	+
7.	Mr. O.	schiz. personal	XXI	+	−
8.	Mr. H.	perversion	XXI	++	+

course of treatment. All except one, Mrs. M., had more than six-month periods of therapy. It should be recalled at this point that telepathic incidents are described as unequivocal when they meet with one or two of the criteria defined in Chapter II. It should also be noted that in the present context chief emphasis was laid on the appearance of tracer elements in the material concerned. The headings "Diagnosis" and "References" are self-explanatory. The plus signs under the headings "Telepathy" indicate one (+) or more (++) telepathic incidents observed. In Table 3 the heading "Therapeutic Response" refers to purely symptomatic, temporary and often deceptive improvements of the clinical picture at the time the telepathic episode occurred. Noting a positive therapeutic response of this order is all that is needed in the present context. But it is needless to say that it must not be mistaken for a claim of effected cure.

Table 4 lists eight controls, taken from a larger number of

TABLE 4

Nr.	Patient	Diagnosis	Ref.: Chapter	Telepathy	Therapeutic Response
1.	Sylvia	compul. neur.	XV	–	+
2.	Mrs. M. L.	compul. neur.	XIV	–	+
3.	Miss R. W.	schizophr.	–	–	+
4.	Mrs. M. B.	anx. hyst.	–	–	+
5.	Mr. G. T.	pervers.	–	–	–
6.	Mrs. N. L.	psychopath.	–	–	+
7.	Mrs. C. Y.	hysteria	–	–	+
8	Mr. G. K.	homosex.	–	–	–

patients treated during the same five-year period. They were selected from about one hundred cases in such a way that their clinical diagnosis, ages, sexes, social status, and cultural backgrounds matched the patients listed in Table 3 in all essential respects. Yet no single incident of overt telepathy was observed in any one of the patients belonging to the control group. It should be further noted that in this group, also, the plus sign under the heading "Therapeutic Response" indicates episodic improvements of the clinical picture observed in apparent response to the usual therapeutic interventions, irrespective of the ultimate outcome of the treatment.

Making allowance for the inaccuracy inherent in such a method of weighing imponderables and measuring largely qualitative data our tabulation should nevertheless make two things perfectly clear. (1) All the eight patients in whom telepathic incidents were observed also showed marked or moderate positive therapeutic responses at the particular time the incident occurred. The only exception from this rule is the schizoid patient listed in Table 3. (2) Table 4, listing eight controls suffering from comparable disorders, shows that similar therapeutic responses were obtained by the same therapist during the same five-year period of observation in the *absence* of overt telepathic incidents.

The reference to "Therapeutic Response" at the particular time the incident occurred needs elucidation. The patient Ruth reported her telepathic dream at a period of marked positive transference which was accompanied by a definite clearing up of hysteric and conversion symptoms and a decrease of her paranoid trend. But for a brief relapse four or five months later the improvement was maintained for three years following termination of therapy.

Ronald H.'s first telepathic dream fell in a period of gradual resolution of neurotic inhibitions and increasing insight into repressed material. A second incident coincided with a dramatic improvement of his sexual adjustment, his ability to work, etc. Within the same week he reported two more presumably telepathic incidents which are not, however, included in the present study.

The occurrence of telepathic incidents in the case of Fred L. marked the turning of the tide of his compulsion neurosis. They were first noted during the tenth, eleventh, and twelfth month of the first period of his treatment. When it was resumed after one year's interval another telepathic dream seemed to usher in a renewed improvement of the clinical picture accompanied by the release of abundant early infantile material.

Mr. T., whose apparently precognitive dream was discussed in Chapters VIII and IX, represents a case of his own. I indicated that the dream occurred at a critical juncture of his treatment. In effect it marked a dramatic improvement of his condition and brought the first break in his obstinate travelling phobia. However, the improvement remained purely symptomatic. The patient failed to make further progress in his analysis. Unable to face his incestuous and pregenital drives which had come into the open he ultimately withdrew from the treatment with his negative transference unresolved and carrying what appeared to be a lasting grudge towards his therapist.

Mrs. M. was seen for a period of two months only, interrupted by a three weeks' stay in a sanatorium during which she received electric shock treatment. Her response to the electric shock was unsatisfactory but had made her at least amenable to subsequent psychotherapy. Her telepathic dream occurred in the fifth week of this second period of psychological treatment while she was still taking barbiturates for sedation. It was during the same week that a definite break seemed to have taken place in her depression. Apart from the evidence of positive transference contained in the dream she showed pronounced interest in the therapist's person, became visibly relaxed, communicative, and gave up some of her hysteric conversion symptoms which complicated the picture. As indicated, however, in Chapter XVII her improvement was short-lived. Four weeks following the telepathic dream psychotherapy had to be discontinued and the patient was admitted to an institution.

In the case of Mr. H., whose dream was described in the previous chapter, the dream itself had occurred in the third week of his treatment. The significant fact is that marked symptomatic improvement of his condition appeared at about the same time. It is undoubtedly to be attributed to the strong positive transference relationship of which the dream itself had been the first indication. It should be noted at this point that the same patient was subsequently involved in a number of telepathic occurrences and that his symptomatic improvement was maintained in the months that followed despite the slow progress made in the dynamic resolution of his conflicts.

Turning to the case of Mr. Z. discussed in Chapter VII it should be recalled that no final judgment was passed as to the true telepathic nature of his "intuitive" anticipation of my thoughts concerning early termination of his treatment. But whatever be the nature of the incident it was accompanied by marked improvement of his condition as well as by added analytic evidence of mastery over his conflicts.

The case of Mr. O., our schizoid writer of science fiction, has been discussed in the previous chapter. He is the patient who produced a distinctly negative response to an apparently trivial telepathic incident although he remained unaware of its telepathic implications. In this case the incident was followed by a brief exacerbation of the patient's condition.

This condensed survey shows that in the first group of cases reviewed here there exists an apparent correlation between telepathic susceptibility on the one hand, and favourable therapeutic response on the other. By and large this apparent correlation duplicates a similar connection between the capacity of establishing a positive transference relationship on the one hand and susceptibility to analytic psychotherapy on the other, well known to psychoanalysts.

* * *

How, then, can this high degree of positive correlation found in our first group of patients be reconciled with the absence of a positive correlation between telepathic susceptibility and therapeutic response in the control group listed in Table 4? I pointed out that this group was composed of patients suffering from a similar set of clinical disorders and showed largely the same tendency to remissions as the group in which unmistakable telepathic incidents have been recorded. I also emphasized that they were undergoing treatment by the same therapist during the same five-year period of his analytic work while he was motivated by identical scientific interests and personality needs.

Yet the apparent inconsistency of our findings is easy to explain. We have to realize that what is here described as the patient's susceptibility to telepathic influences emanating from the therapist has exclusively been determined by reference to tracer elements that made their appearance in his productions. Our first group of patients produced material of just that kind. If in the second group no such tracer elements entered the picture this does not by itself exclude their potential susceptibility on the *psi* level to the therapist's unconscious mental content. It will be recalled that on discussing the telepathic factor involved in both aspects of the transference relationship we have already arrived at exactly the same conclusion. If we are prepared to run the risk attached to all judgments from analogy we may thus be justified in assuming that a positive correlation between telepathic susceptibility and favourable therapeutic response has indeed been in evidence in both groups of patients. Here, again, we may recall Freud's thesis that a similar correlation exists between positive transference and susceptibility to psychotherapy.

But the reader familiar with the elementary principles of the scientific method will rightly object at this point. He may point out that there is a vast difference between so-called positive correlations and the relationship of cause and effect. He may remind us that there is nothing in our material to indicate the way in which telepathy is connected with the improvements observed and that the demonstrability of *psi* in patients showing a positive response to psychotherapy does not justify any conclusions as to the therapeutic value or even therapeutic potentialities of the *psi* factor. Occasional *psi* occurrences or more or less marked susceptibility to telepathy may or may not accompany the patient's positive therapeutic response without, however, being in any way responsible for such a response. He may even hold that telepathy, far from being the cause of improvements achieved, is merely a by-product of the transference relationship, much in the same way as the bacteriologist may find harmless saprophites in water sampled from a famous spa without, however, jumping to the conclusion that its proven curative effect is due to the saprophites found in his sample. In short, the findings reviewed here do not warrant any conclusions as to the actual therapeutic potentialities of the *psi* factor entering the psychoanalytic situation. Its role may be comparable to that of a harmless saprophite thriving wherever conditions are favourable. Alternatively, it may be conducive to some as yet undetected untoward effects, especially in the schizoid personality type. Again, it may, under favourable circumstances, be found to possess undreamt of curative properties comparable to those accidentally discovered in an obscure mould—*Penicillium notatum*. But whether the former or the latter is the case cannot be decided from the bare facts alone which were reviewed in this chapter, and whatever conclusions can be drawn from our comparison of our positive "experimental" cases with the negative "controls" is necessarily of limited value.

Yet it is needless to say that they are by no means the only evidence which is at our disposal. I emphasized in Chapter II that most of the reasoning applied in the field of dynamic psychiatry is based on what I termed the psychological significance of findings, that is, on their consistency with an overall system of rational beliefs. On applying this principle to our observations the assumption of a potential direct therapeutic effect of the *psi* factor is supported by a vast body of collateral evidence derived from various fields of research.

The occasional telepathic activity of the therapist's own unconscious motivations and inner attitudes has been the starting point of our discussion of therapeutic aspects and was described as telepathic leakage. But since there can be little doubt that the wish to help his patient is one of his principal motivations we may rightly conclude that, under favourable circumstances, varying degrees of telepathic activity may be also attached to motivations of this order. More on this point will be said in the chapter that follows.

As far as the potential telepathic effect of such motivations is concerned it is obviously promoted by all the paraphernalia of the psychoanalytic situation. We may only recall the classical rule advising the therapist to meet his patient with an attitude of "suspended attention," without trying to grasp his problem through an active intellectual effort. There is the repudiation of any active interference with the patient's life situation and the rejection of the use of open therapeutic suggestions. There is the warning against excessive therapeutic zeal, whether this be betrayed by the analyst's verbal behaviour or his general attitude in the analytic situation. It is readily understood that, quite apart from psychodynamic considerations, all these injunctions and prohibitions are only apt to reinforce the potential telepathic activity of the analyst's underlying therapeutic motivations.

It is also interesting to note the similarity of the passivity required from the therapist in the analytic situation with certain ancient recipes of how man can avoid suffering and achieve the good life. Lâo-tse, the Chinese mystic of the seventh century B.C., raises his voice in favour of "Wu-Wei," of "deeds without action," while the Hindu philosopher of the same period praises the virtue of full renunciation of worldly desires, a doctrine which is still reflected in Gandhi's precept of non-violence. Again, St. Francis de Sale,[122] nearly one millennium after his Far Eastern predecessors, reminds the faithful of the birds who are only caught in nets and snares "because they move and struggle immoderately to escape from them and in doing so entangle themselves so much more." He calls on his disciples to "place their spirits in a state of tranquillity and repose, calming their judgment and will."

Similar exhortations can be found in teachings of many religious leaders, mystics, and philosophers, ancient and modern, Western and Oriental. Clearly, their resemblance to Freud's[44i] precept asking for the passivity of the analyst cannot be accidental. They are based on age-old experience in trying to allay human suffering—whether this be sought in the shadow of a mango tree, in the quiet of a medieval church or on the analyst's couch. And even though the principle of Wu-Wei were of negative survival value in the rough and tumble of everyday life it still serves an important purpose in the narrow sector reserved for psychotherapy in our culture.

Viewed from our angle it may well be the therapist's inhibited impulse to take action or even to verbalize suppressed therapeutic suggestions which serves as a decisive aid in getting them "across" to the patient on the *psi* level. It will be recalled that in all experiments of the ESP type attempts at deliberate and premeditated telepathic agency were doomed to failure, and success depended largely on the relaxed and spontaneous attitude of both agent and percipient.

The "basic rule" which the patient is called upon to observe in the psychoanalytic situation is also in good keeping with rhis general principle. The emphasis on free associations, on tenunciation of all volitional effort to bring up "relevant" material are all designed to relax conscious control. Yet in so doing it facilitates not only the emergence of repressed autopsychic material but also enhances susceptibility to heteropsychic influences.

Another important predisposing factor is represented by a special aspect of the transference relationship to which little reference has been made so far in our argument. We know that the patient, whenever he develops a marked transference to the therapist, is apt to re-enact some of his early childhood conflicts in relation to his parents. In so doing he tends to regress to the infantile level and actually to exhibit behaviour patterns pertaining to that stage. Now even though this regression may affect only a limited segment of the patient's personality it may amount to a new opening for the analyst's therapeutic approach. In Chapter XIII I discussed in some detail the infant's striking susceptibility to infinitesimal clues transmitted to him from his mother on the ego, the id, and the *psi* level. These influences, I stated, have a profound effect upon the whole development of the child, upon the moulding of his social character and his acculturation. Much the same considerations apply to the patient's attitude in relation to his therapist. He, too, may under conditions of marked positive transference develop a heightened susceptibility to both sensory and non-sensory clues emanating from the analyst which may then play an important part in the therapeutic process.

I mentioned the case of the infant who, induced by the coprophilic attitudes of his mother, develops an exaggerated interest in his excretions and may actually resort to coprophagia. I quoted the case of little May who refused to eat the "nice liver soup" offered to her by an aunt only because the child seemed to "sense" the latter's indiosyncrasy about the "insides of animals." We saw how little Anne fulfilled in her neurotic behaviour the unconscious wishes and expectations of her mother, while at the same time defying the latter's commands expressed on the verbal level.

It is from observations of this kind that we arrived at the conclusion that telepathic influences passing both ways between mother and child are responsible for much more than occasional frictions between the two. They may play a significant part in controlling the child's emotional growth, social adjustment, and acculturation in general.

This picture of the three-level relationship between parent and child, as it was described in Chapter XIII, can serve as a simplified model of the relationship between therapist and patient. This relationship can be conceived as a re-enactment by the patient of early childhood attitudes in which he is ready to respond to infinitesimal clues communicated to him by the analyst on the ego, the id, and *psi* level, while the analyst himself may enhance the patient's response by the self-imposed restraint of his tendency to vicarious functioning on his behalf. To put it in other words: the therapist's enkinetic attitude, seasoned and matured by his analytic training, may meet halfway the patient's empathic response the ground for which has already been prepared by the whole analytic situation and particularly by the transference relationship.

We have seen that under favourable circumstances the patient's reactions to three-level influences of this order are indeed surprisinglystrong. Sometimes they seem to approximate to the infant's ready response to unverbalized commands, wishes, and expectations transmitted to him by his mother. It may well be that some of the proven techniques of analytical psychotherapy—including the outer paraphernalia of the analytic situation—have inadvertently been developed so as to serve just that purpose.

All these considerations go far to show that telepathy, far from being a mere by-product of the psychotherapeutic approach, may indeed serve as an important aid in conveying to the patient the therapist's unverbalized therapeutic motivations. Provided that he approaches his task with the "right kind" of therapeutic motivations, it may thus become an integral part of the therapeutic process itself. It is to this aspect of the psychoanalytic situation that we will turn our attention in the next chapter.

CHAPTER XXIII

How is the Therapist Involved?

A Digression into the Dynamics of Co-operation

THERE are few areas of interpersonal relationships in which three-level analysis is of greater significance—and perhaps more rewarding—than the therapist's relationship to his patient. Obviously the attitudes indicated by the Hippocratic Oath, by the code of Maimonides* or by the parable of the Good Samaritan scratch the surface only. Psychoanalysis, probing below the surface, has revealed some of the motivating forces which operate on deeper levels of the therapist's personality. It has shown that the physician, being a human, may use his profession in a quest for magic control or omnipotence over his environment. G. Róheim[106a] traced this attitude back to the primitive medicine man. He described his ritualistic practices as sublimated products of underlying sadistic impulses directed against what had originally been the victims of "black magic." In Róheim's view vestiges of similar attitudes can still be found in the modern counterpart of the primitive witch doctor.

E. Simmel[115] sees similar attitudes reflected in the "doctor game" which is so frequently played by children in our culture. He suggests that in this game the child, playing the part of the surgeon armed with the "big knife," impersonates the role ascribed to the cruel father in the primal scene. A patient of mine, a woman of thirty-nine, liked to cut up frogs, lizards, and caterpillars as a child of eight years. Charlie, the neighbour's son, was the leader in this game. Charlie is a noted

* "May the love for my art actuate me at all times. May neither avarice nor miserliness nor the thirst for glory nor for a great reputation engage my mind."
MOSES MAIMONIDES.

surgeon today while my patient made nursing her career. Observations like these indicate that the surgeon of our days may indeed select his speciality so as to divert a latent sadistic trend into socially more desirable channels. L. Szondi[126] has come out with a great number of genealogical data derived from his studies in *Fate Analysis* in support of such a thesis. Psychoanalytically speaking, choosing the medical profession may be the outcome of elaborate reaction formations to self-seeking, egotistic tendencies; or else it may constitute a paradoxical blend of highly sublimated reaction formations and the perfectly legitimate need for attaining the social standing and financial rewards which go with it.

B. V. Strauss,[124] in a recent article, specifically listed prestige hunger, the need to be authoritative, to be omniscient, to "do good," to be loved—or else to rule and to dominate, as some of the common unconscious motivations of the physician and called attention to their harmful effect, so long as they pass unnoticed, upon the doctor-patient relationship. Such attitudes may cause blind spots in the therapist's approach to his patients and make him overly indulgent or less tolerant of some of their complaints or personality traits.

The discovery of what I described as telepathic leakage has revealed other motivations, largely unconscious, which may play an important part in the therapist's approach. In effect, most examples of telepathic tracer effects upon which our argument is based are due to motivations of which the therapist has originally been unaware and which are accidental to the purpose of the treatment. Even though there is nothing sinister about motivations of this kind, their potential telepathic activity upon the mind of the patient confronts us with a momentous question. We have to ask: in what way, if any, can the therapist bring only the therapeutically desirable aspects of his motivations to bear upon his patients while suppressing therapeutically indifferent or frankly undesirable motivations? Is the therapist's training analysis, with its ruthless exposure of his narcissistic, sadistic or otherwise neurotic attitudes, the answer to the question—or has he to resign himself, with Shakespeare's King Richard II, that neither analysis nor water can wash away his sins, and leave his professional eligibility to the Grace of God or the Calvinist principle of Election? Is there no escape from what the theologian Paul Tillich[128] has called man's "possession from below" and has he no option but to pin his hope on its dialectical opposite: "possession from above"?

Psychoanalysis has made allowance for this problem by studying the therapist's countertransference on his patient. Originally it sought to impose a strict ban on any and every kind of emotional involvement by the analyst in the treatment relationship. But it was soon found that such an attitude cannot possibly be maintained in practice. The analyst cannot help responding in one way or another to the emotional aspects of the psychoanalytical situation. But in doing so he is called upon to recognize his reactions and to use them for the benefit of the treatment.

Anni Reich,[99] in a recent article, has pointed out that Freud's plea for a completely unemotional attitude of the therapist does not mean that he has to remain nothing but a screen upon which his patient should project his emotional conflicts. Although the therapist may occasionally misuse his countertransference for purposes alien to the analytic situation a "slight shift in cathexis" may transform an unconscious mechanism of the analyst from "a living out of his own conflicts into a valuable sublimation."

In a similar vein, Margaret Little[75] holds that analysis must become a "true sublimation for the analyst, not an emotional outlet for his neurotic needs or a defence against his phobic or paranoid attitudes" which may easily be sensed by the patient. Statements like these reflect the general trend of thinking about the problem of countertransference in current psychoanalytic literature.

But what happens when the therapist fails to achieve a "true sublimation" of his undesirable unconscious motivations? What are the factors in his personality which should outweigh or counteract the untoward effects of his hostile or self-seeking impulses brought to bear upon his patient on the *psi* level? In short, what is the nature of the ultimate driving forces which make true co-operation between therapist and patient for a common purpose possible after all?

The question, formulated in this way, is begging the answer. It is influenced by preconceived ideas about the depravity of human nature, and more specifically by Darwin's[25] theory of evolution with its emphasis on competition and the combative instinct. Yet Darwin himself never denied that dependence of one being on another may itself have positive survival value. This thesis was further elaborated by the Russian anarchist and biologist Kropotkin[72] who expressly pleaded for the recognition of mutual aid as an important factor in evolution. More recent experimental observations by W. M. Wheeler,[136] M. C. Allee[4] and many others have placed Kropotkin's somewhat amateurish theories on more secure scientific foundations. Professor Allee has pointed out that in addition to the well-known self-centred egotistic drives, group-centred, more or less altruistic drives are an integral feature of interaction among animals. They are responsible for what he describes as unconscious or automatic interaction and interdependence in nature. Earlier observations in the field of experimental social psychology dealing with the part played by co-operation versus competition in human societies point in the same direction (Gardner Murphy and T. M. Newcomb[86c]).

Unfortunately, psychoanalysis has failed, so far, to support the findings of the ecologists and biologically oriented sociologists. Focusing, as it does, attention upon the untramelled instinctual drives of the id, it finds ample evidence of hostility and aggression and is inclined to describe what evidence of fellowship, humanitarian and philanthropic attitudes can be observed in man's mental make-up in terms of sublimations, reaction formations or masochistic tendencies.

But paying due attention to the two basic attitudes of empathy and enkinesis we hit upon what might easily prove to be the very physiological roots of man's sense of solidarity and co-operation with his fellow-men. Empathy and enkinesis, we said, are direct derivatives from such common neurological mechanisms as ill-defined protopathic perceptions in the sensory field and loosely co-ordinated synergistic movements in the motor sphere. They are to be considered as direct extensions into the heteropsychic sphere of our autopsychic sensory and motor functioning. They are the means by which, psychoanalytically speaking, the ego is capable of extending its cathexis from its own confines to the non-ego.

Once the power of these two basic tendencies of the ego is properly understood there should be no difficulty in reconciling the findings of modern biology with our new and expanded concept of personality.

The physiological roots of Allee's[4] unconscious co-operation and interdependence in human society obviously lie in the very nature of man's ego organization. Man's concern for his fellows is nothing but a direct continuation of his concern for himself. On a deeper level it is based on his intrinsic need to re-establish, if only in a functional way, his lost solidarity with his fellow-men. Co-operation is thus not a dictate from outside. It is the corollary of his biological make-up which makes him an integral part of the family group and the community at large, even though the bonds connecting him with them may not be visible to the naked eye. It is a basic function of the ego and like many other ego functions frequently unconscious. Co-operation between man and his fellows, between parent and child, between therapist and patient, is thus a function inherent in our neuro-biological organization. To be sure, it need not necessarily be called into action whenever it is needed but it is one among many potentialities of human behaviour subject to deliberate encouragement and cultivation—or repression and progressive functional atrophy, as the case may be.

The psychoanalytic concept of identification, transference or countertransference covers only one aspect of this attitude. It rather amounts to the consummation in the social sphere of the tendency to "imaginative projection of our consciousness" into another person's sensory experience and its counterpart, the tendency to imaginative sharing of motor attitudes directed at coping with danger situations and emergencies that threaten the life and the well-being of the individual.

Needless to say, there is an infinite number of derivatives from this basic ego function. They range from the magic wish for omnipotence on one end to the highly sublimated attitude of compassion, sympathy, and universal fellowship, or the ancient Hindu doctrine of *tatwam asi,* on the other end of the scale. There is the possessive mother holding on to her offspring as though it was a direct continuation of her own personality. There is the power-hungry dictator striving to bring a nation, and if possible the whole world, under his control. There is the proselytizing religious fanatic who seeks to lift the same expansionist drive to a purportedly spiritual plane. And there is the cold, calculating fervour of the scientist who aims at bringing the entire universe of facts and figures under an all-embracing unified system of thought.

Clearly, the psychiatrist, approaching his patient as a helper in his plight, is animated by derivatives of similar personality needs. Indeed, in his case the connection between the basic need of the ego for extension into the non-ego and the tendency to empathic sharing and vicarious functioning is much more direct and obvious. It is a derivative blended in part from the attitude of the controlling parent, in part from that of the primitive medicine man in quest of omnipotence, tempered by the attitude of the scientist striving for knowledge and intellectual mastery over his social and physical environment. Yet under whatever flag his attitude may sail, whatever cultural guise it may assume, his basic motivations—like that of the physician in general—is derived from his original sense of solidarity with his fellow-men and his intrinsic tendency to function vicariously on their behalf.

* * *

However, the mere fact that a definite socially oriented empathic and enkinetic trend can be discerned in man's mental organization does not by itself indicate that it must necessarily assert itself and determine overt behaviour in the give and take of everyday life. We may possess the capacity of reaching out by imaginative projection to our fellow-men but this does not guarantee by any means that we are bound or even prepared to make use of this capacity in a given social situation. Nor does it automatically cancel out all the undercurrents of hostility and aggression which continue to exist on deeper levels. This is equally true for the treatment situation as for interpersonal relationships in general.

In the last analysis our impact upon our fellows is determined by goals and purposes that motivate the personality as a whole, that is, by the integration of attitudes stemming from the ego, the id, and the *psi* level, with all the uncertainties that integration of controllable and uncontrollable elements implies. Indeed, to the extent to which uncontrollable elements are involved in the psychotherapeutic situation it cannot be denied that it still falls short of the status of a strictly rational scientific procedure.

CHAPTER XXIV

Scientific Psychotherapy and the Decline of Magic

THE intrinsic difficulties of exercising control over the primitive aspects of the therapist's personality—of making his unconscious fall in line with the major strategy of the treatment—are an embarrassing conclusion from our argument. Psychotherapy, conceived as a rational scientific procedure, presupposes two things: first, full knowledge of all the factors involved and, secondly, mastery over these factors. I indicated that only to the extent to which psychotherapy has achieved this end can it claim to be a strictly scientific discipline. To the extent to which it falls short of this objective it is still burdened by its ancient legacy of magic.

Yet it is just such observations as described here which indicate that modern dynamic psychiatry, despite its avowed scientific aspirations, has not been able to make a complete break from its primitive, pre-scientific past. Indeed, it may well be that it is precisely its excessive iconoclastic zeal which has hampered the dispassionate study of the broken idols, leaving a vast gap in our understanding of the magic substrata of the human mind. The result is an uncompromisingly rationalistic system of thought which owes its very consistency to a scientifically self-defeating omission.

Yet, however embarrassing this may be, modern psychiatry cannot deny its derivation from the magic art of healing of a bygone age. There undoubtedly is a straight line of descent from the ritualistic practices of the primitive witch-doctor to the more sophisticated methods used by Mesmer in the eighteenth century, or by Dr. Braid of Manchester, to Charcot and Liebeault and to the early experiments with hypnoanalysis carried out by Breuer and Freud at the turn of the nineteenth century. In the course of this development the magic, pre-scientific element more and more receded into the background and the rational techniques of scientific psychotherapy gained increasing prominence, a trend which ultimately reached its consummation in the later stages of the classical Freudian doctrine. On the face of it modern psychoanalytic theory has indeed succeeded in making a clean sweep of the last vestiges of magic that were left in earlier systems and in bringing the methods of psychological treatment as close to the standard of a rationally conceived and executed scientific procedure as could possibly be attained in the psychological sphere. (See Fig. 13.)

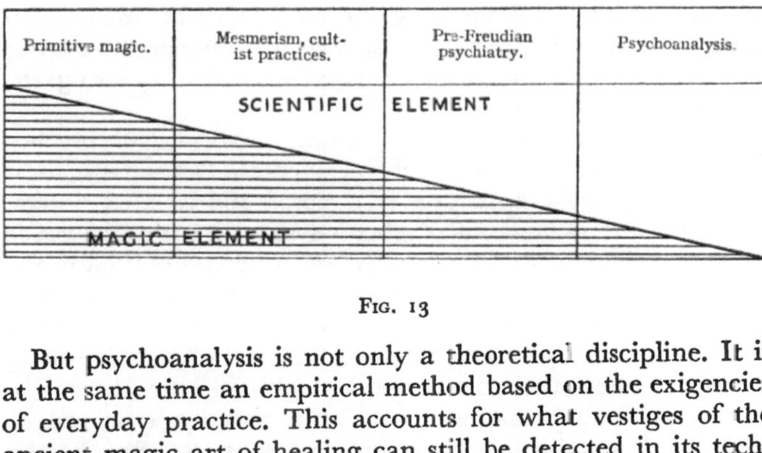

FIG. 13

But psychoanalysis is not only a theoretical discipline. It is at the same time an empirical method based on the exigencies of everyday practice. This accounts for what vestiges of the ancient magic art of healing can still be detected in its technique. We may only recall the outer paraphernalia of the psychoanalytic situation to which we have already referred in Chapter XXII. Their avowed purpose is the mobilization of repressed unconscious material. But their resemblance to certain cultist observances is unmistakable. There is the emphasis on the patient's relaxed, reclining position—a remnant of certain Yogi practices or of the Temple Sleep of the ancients and of the bodily posture thought to be conducive to Mesmeric trance. There is the admonition addressed to the patient to renounce all volitional efforts; to avoid organizing his thoughts in a rational way and thereby to facilitate the flow of free associations. Again, there is the rule advising the therapist to assume much the same passive, relaxed attitude, to meet his patient in a state of "suspended attention," giving free rein to his own unconscious, and to refrain from trying to grasp his problem on the intellectual level only. There is the exercise of what Bernard Shaw has called the "appropriate austerities" which seems to be mandatory on both saints and psychoanalysts—and there is, above all, the tendency of the patient himself to give a magic connotation to the therapist's role in the treatment situation.

We know that all these empirical rules and outer paraphernalia of psychoanalytic technique do in effect serve their purpose. But we have seen that they also have an important side effect: besides facilitating the emergence of unconscious material from the autopsychic sphere they loosen the barrier which blocks the way to heteropsychic material entering the confines of the ego.

Yet if such is the effect of certain provisions of psychoanalytic technique it is purely accidental. Conceiving as it does of the psychic apparatus as a closed and isolated system, the conceptual scheme of psychoanalysis makes no allowance for the possible operation of *psi*. Its theory confines itself to the study of such psychic agencies as the ego, the super-ego, and the id. It allows for the modification of instinctual drives which reside in the id by raising them to the level of consciousness; it seeks to effect their discharge through cathartic abreaction or gradual transformation into higher, socially approved or sublimated activities, and so on and so forth. But in the absence of the requisite neural pathways it cannot admit the possibility of anything like a direct action by one unconscious upon another unconscious, and where it is forced by actual clinical experience to make such an assumption it does so only in a figurative manner of speaking, e.g. by reference to unknown factors operating in the personality of the therapist.

In the previous chapter we have sought to arrive at a better understanding of these unknown personality factors. We tried to indicate the presumable telepathic effect of the physician's unconscious therapeutic motivations and countertransference upon his patient. But it is still a far cry from this insight to the control and systematic utilization and development of the *psi* factor in the framework of planned scientific psychotherapy. *Psi* functions are subject to what I described as the principle of frustrated volition. They are difficult to cultivate in our present cultural setting and generally defy the familiar methods of training and education provided in our Western colleges and universities. Their acquisition has been compared to the learning of such highly specialized skills as playing a musical instrument, becoming proficient in the use of the differential calculus or to becoming a champion at chess. But there are two basic differences between *psi* functions and teachable skills of the ordinary kind which should not be overlooked. First, the range of *psi* functions extends beyond the confines of the auto-psychic sphere; secondly neither the functions themselves nor their motivating forces are accessible to the therapist's deliberate volition. These are difficulties no violinist, mathematician or chess player has to contend with.

We have to realize, moreover, that any attempt at cultivating *psi* abilities by focusing attention upon the performance of a few prize subjects in ESP would miss the point. We have to realize that *psi* is not an independent function at all. The available evidence rather indicates that *psi* elements are woven into a wide variety of ego functions and are intimately blended with what we described as empathic and enkinetic attitudes in everyday life. They are part of our ordinary mental functioning and neither "sub-normal," "para-normal" nor "super-normal."

One is reminded at this point of the way in which several levels of the central nervous system work together in the adaptive behaviour of the organism. We know that both cortical, i.e. pyramidal, and subcortical, i.e. extrapyramidal, centres are involved in the control of our muscular system. Likewise, it is the fusion of so-called epicritic and protopathic stimuli received from outside (and inside) the body and processed in cortical and subcortical centres of the brain which is involved in the making of our perceptual world. We know, furthermore, that in the case of pyramidal lesions the remaining extrapyramidal functions are basically inaccessible to the patient's spontaneous volition and can only be mobilized under the influence of strong affect. Similar conclusions have to be drawn from studies of so-called protopathic sensory functions controlled by thalamic centres of the brain.

But if our comparison is justified we are led back once more to our original question: how, then, can the *psi* factor contained in the therapist's enkinetic attitude, that is, a function barely reaching the standard of poorly co-ordinated extra-pyramidal motor impulses (or the level of vaguely perceived thalamic sensations) be so trained, disciplined, and refined as to make it suitable for such highly skilled and specialized operations as those involved in psychotherapy?

To find the answer to this question we have to revert to the observations discussed in the first part of this book. These observations show that although most incidents described were of a spontaneous nature—and not the result of the therapist's or the patient's deliberate volition—they came about in response to certain personality needs of those involved. More often than not they were elicited by certain situational stresses, social demands or pressures affecting the therapist. As far as the present writer is concerned an important predisposing factor should be noted at this point. His early observations which served as eye openers, as it were, in his case date from the time of his war-time exile in England. They were made at a period when more than his personal safety and economic security were endangered and the need for adjustment to a new environment had reached a critical stage of urgency. It is possible that such recurrent themes as his home and other earthly possessions as are contained in his patients' telepathic productions owe their special emotional significance to this state of affairs. These items had become detached parts of the therapist's extended body image, as it were. Like the phantom limb of an amputee they became invested with extra cathexis or emotional interest.

Some of the observations recorded by Pederson-Krag,[93] J. Meerloo[81] and E. Servadio[112] point in the same direction. Pederson-Krag's patients, for instance, seemed to reflect in their telepathic productions anxiety-laden problems of her own, seeking to allay, at the same time, anxieties common to both therapist and patient. The same is true for the telepathic incidents described in Chapters IV and V. Again, one of

Jule Eisenbud's[33a] most striking examples of telepathy was precipitated by his own need to defend his case and hold his own in a bitter scientific controversy.

What, then, is the lesson that can be learned from observations of this kind? They indicate that anxiety, generated by stressful life situations, deflected from aggressive outlets and channelized by an unusual set of cultural demands, may bring forth reactions which are not otherwise elicited in response to the ordinary stimuli, social cues, and incentives which determine behaviour on the ego level. This is illustrated by the very fact that some of the incidents described here were stimulated by the emotional interest of those involved in the subject-matter of telepathy itself. But if this is true it can well be assumed that a shift of emphasis from motivations *extraneous* to the treatment to the *real thing*, i.e. to the overriding remedial purpose of the psychoanalytic situation, may result in an "operant reinforcement" of the therapist's unconscious wishes and expectations in the direction of *therapeutic responses* in preference to a few striking but therapeutically indifferent tracer effects.

We know that highly charged life situations, environmental pressures and penalizations have always served as powerful incentives for cultural change. Professor A. Toynbee's[130] theory of the historic process is largely based upon this fundamental proposition. The history of medicine abounds with examples of high achievement among members of disintegrating civilizations. The celebrated healers of the late Hellenistic period, the great physicians of the declining Islamic world, are cases in point, to say nothing of the contributions of Jewish and other minority groups to the progress of psychological medicine in particular.

There are in this way three principal factors which combine in bringing about the specific psychological configuration needed for the mobilization of *psi* functions for psychotherapy: (1) situations of stress affecting the therapist's attitude towards his calling on a deep level; (2) his single-minded devotion to a cause—in our case to the cause of *psi*-level therapy itself, and, (3) a general atmosphere of approbation prevailing within the group in which he is called upon to operate.

Bringing about a psychological constellation of this order certainly is a task that goes beyond the capacities of the individual therapist. But even if some of its ingredients are of a basically uncontrollable nature they no longer fall within the province of magic. The psychiatrist, at the present stage, is much in the same position as the surgeon of a past era, who was engaged in the treatment of wounds and wound infections unaware of the host of micro-organisms whose presence was apt to influence, for better or for worse, the recovery of his patients. In the psychiatrist's case the newly discovered agent is the *psi* factor entering the analytic situation. Its proper appreciation—and ultimate control—may well usher in a new era in the advancement of psychotherapy comparable to that opened up in the field of surgery by the nineteenth-century discovery of bacteriology.

CHAPTER XXV

Some Principles and Problems of Three-Level Therapy

WHAT, then, are the therapeutic implications of the *psi* factor involved in the psychoanalytic situation? In what way, if any, can it be integrated with our current analytic approach to ego and id levels and become an adjunct of proven therapeutic techniques? Needless to say, all attempts at doing so are still in their infancy. At the present juncture we can do little more than formulate some of the problems which present themselves on our way and lay down certain principles which have already proved their usefulness in our work.

There is, first, the eminently practical question whether or not the telepathic nature of an incident observed in the psychoanalytic situation should be disclosed to the patient. And if so, at what stage of the treatment should this be done? All the evidence available so far indicates that interpretations involving *psi* incidents should only be given at an advanced stage of analysis, when all aspects of the transference relationship have been thoroughly worked through and when the therapist feels safe to expose whatever evidence of his own counter-transference is contained in the telepathic material under review. Even so its disclosure may put the transference relationship to a severe test and supply the patient with new material to rationalize his resistance to the treatment.

The risks involved in such disclosures should not, however, be over-estimated. We must not forget that on the *psi* level all analytic work is carried out in a glass house, as it were, with the therapist's unconscious constantly exposed to the telepathic scrutiny of his patient. Indeed, an analyst who feels he cannot afford to be seen and to go about his job under such conditions had better disqualify himself from his professional work. He has to realize that, however impersonal and detached his approach on the ego level may be, he cannot possibly prevent his patient from responding to his unconscious inner attitudes and motivations. But I have stressed that under favourable circumstances it is this very fact which may also serve as a valuable tool of the treatment. If properly timed, the frank discussion of the therapist's *psi*-level involvement in the transference relationship may serve as an opening wedge for the emergence of dissociated mental content which the patient himself might otherwise be unable to face.

The results obtained with this procedure have been encouraging so far. Yet a note of caution has to be sounded at this point. Although I mentioned that as a general rule marked negative transference militates against the emergence of *psi*, any reference to the occurrence of telepathy has to be carefully avoided under such conditions. This is particularly true for the advanced schizophrenic who may easily use interpretations involving *psi* factors as added confirmation of his delusional trend. On the other hand due allowance made for the patient's direct susceptibility to the therapist's unconscious or preconscious mental content is nowhere more rewarding than in the case of the schizophrenic. The early schizophrenic is particularly sensitive to influences of this kind. He is allergic, as it were, to the slightest indication of attempted control transmitted to him by the therapist's demeanour—on whatever level such impressions may be conveyed to him. But he can be counted on to open up and relax his defences once he is reassured by genuine detachment and restraint on the part of the therapist.

A second problem encountered in three-level therapy as conceived here refers to the utilization of insight afforded by the telepathic material. I have repeatedly stated in previous chapters that such material should be treated in exactly the same manner as material derived from the autopsychic sphere. The way in which the very fact of its emergence may influence the dynamic evaluation of a given situation is another question. As a general rule it testifies to an intimate *psi*-level *rapport* between therapist and patient, even under circumstances in which other clues to that effect have not as yet been forthcoming. In many cases, I said, it is the proper appreciation of a telepathic element contained in the patient's productions which closes the gap in the understanding of a neurotic symptom, a faulty action or a dream reported by the patient. Its telepathic interpretation will then depend on the considerations mentioned above, as well as on the criteria which apply to the giving of interpretations in general.

This leads to a third question, touching on one of the most problematic aspects of therapeutic technique: to the question of interpretation as a tool of psychoanalytic therapy. It may be well to distinguish between two sides of the problem. Interpretation involves, first, a full dynamic understanding by the therapist of the patient's conflicts, of his personality structure, of the nature of his ego defences at a given time, and so on and so forth. Equally important is a second point: the patient's readiness to accept the interpretation offered to him and his ability to assimilate the insight gained with the rest of his personality.

As a general rule there is a considerable time-lag between these two phases of interpretation. The therapist may have attained far-reaching understanding, e.g., of the latent meaning of a symptom, but it may be a matter of months before he feels safe to convey this insight to his patient. Yet we have to realize that this period of abstinence and self-imposed restraint, however strictly adhered to, may have the diametrically opposite effect on the *psi* level. I emphasized that it is precisely attitudes of this kind which may, under favourable conditions, promote telepathic activity. If this is true there must be a more or less prolonged period in every analytic treatment during which the patient is exposed to subliminal *psi* influences emanating from the therapist prior to the verbal communication of the same content on the ego level. Put in other words, one could say: verbal interpretations are usually preceded by a period of incubation during which they may or may not be tacitly registered on the *psi* level. If properly timed, verbal interpretations may then act as reinforcements of whatever previous effects they may have had on the *psi* level.

It is readily understood that this state of affairs may at times become a serious pitfall to the validity of the interpretations themselves. In Chapter XX, dealing with the problem of telepathic leakage, I have already pointed out that such leakage may decisively influence the patient's productions at any stage of the treatment. Telepathic leakage may do this in one of two ways. First, the interpretation may amount to a correct dynamic evaluation of the case but is, nevertheless, largely based on material derived from telepathic leakage. It may then lead to what can be described as a situation of *simulated authenticity* in which the patient seems to obey all the rules of the "game," in which all the hypothetical layers of his genetic personality structure are being expertly exposed, and all his developmental stages worked through in the proper order—yet his therapeutic response may be slight, and what improvement he shows may be largely due to suggestion. Alternatively, the interpretation may be exclusively based on telepathic leakage and reflect nothing but the therapist's own preconceived ideas and theoretical expectations. Spurious interpretations of this type are either completely ineffective or may only increase the patient's resistance. They may then result in what Wilhelm Reich[100] has described as *chaotic situations* in psychoanalysis and lead to complete therapeutic failure.

There is no use denying the difficulties arising from this state of affairs. The therapist failing to realize the pitfalls of telepathic leakage may find himself in the position of a child caught in a maze conjured up by mirrors mounted on opposite walls. He may mistake his own reflection for another person confronting him on the other side of the looking glass. He may be gratified to see all his theories vindicated by his patients, whereas in effect their productions amount to nothing but renewed confirmation of the fact of telepathic leakage, aided, maybe, by veiled or overt suggestion.

There is, however, one point to remember which tends to diminish the ambiguity created by the occurrence of telepathic leakage. Although it is true to say that it may bring out material derived from the therapist's rather than from the patient's unconscious we have seen in the first part of this book that the very occurrence of telepathy is itself facilitated by the presence of identical dynamic configurations (repressed "complexes," emotional conflicts, etc.) of those involved. Conversely, the absence of such common ground seems to militate against telepathic leakage and against the emergence of telepathy in general.

All this shows once more that on the *psi* level strict discrimination between the patient's and the therapist's contribution to a specific phase of analytic insight is not really necessary nor indeed possible. We have to assume that on this level the two cease to operate as two closed and isolated personality units. They rather merge into a new functional system in its own right based on the community of their analytic experience. In fact, what is often described as an occasional flash of telepathic communication between two separate individuals is nothing more than a manifestation of their temporary functional unity on the *psi* level which happens to ripple the surface of the ego.

Seen from this angle the question as to the actual source or ownership of unconscious material that makes its appearance at a particular stage of analysis is no longer of decisive importance. The important point is the very fact of its emergence and the emotional repercussions which follow in the wake of such an event. Neither is the language in which the actual interpretation is couched of major importance. It may make use of Freudian, Jungian or Adlerian symbolism or of more or less private idioms or figures of speech. On a deeper level their meaning is the same. In the last analysis an interpretation is nothing but a stimulus striking the patient on the ego level but filtering down to unconscious strata and setting in motion a chain of events which, if skilfully handled, ultimately result in a dynamic change of personality in the desired direction. As in the broader field of sensory perception this effect is largely independent of the nature of the stimulus itself and is determined by what Johannes Müller called the specific energies of the receptor organs—in our case, by the specific configurations in the id upon which it impinges.

Theoretically speaking it is conceivable that in an extreme case an effective interpretation is imparted on the patient without the aid of verbal communication although its effect can greatly be enhanced if proper verbalization secures participation of the patient's personality on the ego level.

R. Loewenstein,[76] discussing the importance of verbalizing in psychoanalytic treatment, has rightly pointed out that spoken words are social realities which may profoundly affect the patient's personality as a whole.

The community of emotional experience to both patient and therapist which is implied by dynamically valid interpretations calls for one more word of comment. Obviously, there are two sides of the picture which have to be considered, one pertaining to the therapist, the other to the patient. As in a two-colour print its component parts are in effect derived from both parties. George Devereux,[27] in a recent article, compares the patient's productions over the whole period of analysis with fragments of a jigsaw puzzle which gradually suggest a meaningful pattern or Gestalt to the therapist. Once all the fragments are brought into the open and the last missing piece of information falls into place what Gestalt psychologists call a tension system may reach the point of closure, thus satisfying a "need" inherent in the system. Certainly, this formulation covers but one aspect of the process. But it serves as a graphic description of the dynamics of interpretation in terms of Gestalt psychology. Also, it is equally applicable to the therapist whose tension system has, as a general rule, been of much longer standing than that of his patient and has been subject to brief or intermittent phases of "closure" only. Put in terms of Gestalt psychology one could say that on the *psi* level there are no such things as separate tension systems pertaining to patient or therapist respectively. Neither is the question as to which of the two supplied the missing fragment to the jigsaw puzzle needed to complete the Gestalt of any real importance. Important is the formation of a shared pattern of emotional experience itself, bringing about, though for a fleeting moment only, a functional unity of the two.

The psychodynamic significance of such an experience cannot possibly be over-estimated. There is nothing lonelier in the universe than a fully self-contained and isolated ego whose emotional contact with his social environment has been blocked by the growing self-sufficiency demanded by our culture or obliterated by an existing mental disorder. I indicated in Chapter XVII that all our efforts to evolve many and varied systems of communication with our fellow-man, from person to person and from group to group, only serve the purpose of mitigating or making up for the cosmic loneliness of the individual in our Western civilization. In fact the gregarious patterns of all types of human association, from the family to the clan, from the Firemen's Mutual Benefit Association to the State and the United Nations, are so designed as to restore in a functional way the lost solidarity of the individual with the rest of the world.

The community of experience which can be achieved at certain points of psychoanalytic treatment seems to be a short cut in this direction. It may result in a re-enactment and re-living on the *psi* level of man's original solidarity with his species, represented by parental figures—and their symbolic substitute: the therapist. For the patient it may amount to the consummation in the transference relationship of a desire common to all humanity: to go back to one's point of departure and to make a fresh start in life once again.

Another important aspect of psychoanalytic technique which is directly affected by our approach is that of planning. The problem of planning is automatically involved in the therapist's diagnostic and prognostic considerations of his case. These considerations can in turn hardly be dissociated from his tacit expectation of failure or success, with all its potential repercussions on the *psi* level upon the patient. Indeed there is reason to believe that the therapist's preconscious anticipation of the course likely to be taken by the treatment may itself influence its final outcome. So far as the gradual attainment of the goals of therapy is concerned it is perhaps impossible to draw a sharp demarcation line between the arrival at a diagnosis, the proper appraisal of existing therapeutic possibilities, the anticipation of results and the operation on the *psi* level of the therapist's enkinetic and empathic attitudes, carrying within themselves the seed of their self-fulfilment.

Here, again, we are reminded of our original model of the psychoanalytic situation: the child-parent relationship. We have to assume that on the *psi* level the therapist's approach to his patient is nothing but a duplication of a parent's eager anticipation of his child's natural growth and development.

But in the therapist's case this approach is guided at the same time by his intimate knowledge of the patient's emotional disturbance, his inner resources and potentialities. If he be equal to his task, his therapeutic motivations and inner attitudes will be oriented towards what areas of unimpaired growth are still left in the patient. On the other hand he will also be aware of his limitations. He will know that he has to refrain from any direct attack upon such fixed phobic, compulsive or delusional symptoms which in his estimate are beyond his reach at the particular phase of the treatment—and he will seek to maintain this attitude of non-intervention not only on the ego but also on the *psi* level. It goes without saying that he will likewise make a point of abstaining on all levels of his personality from attempts at active therapeutic intervention under conditions of negative transference and in negativistic patients in general. An overly eager, ambitious therapist is bound to provoke resistance in any type of patient comparable to the patterns of resisting habitually provoked by over-solicitous or compulsive parents in their offspring.

Viewed from our angle the long-term strategy of the treatment proceeds in three principal stages. In the opening phases the therapist may be aided by *psi* factors, particularly by his empathic response to his patient's personality. This period imperceptibly merges into and overlaps with a second phase in which the emphasis shifts to more or less explicit therapeutic expectations and enkinetic attitudes. A third phase may be reserved for verbalization of insights gained, working through processes and for the resolution of the transference relationship, according to proven precepts of current analytic techniques. But it is needless to say that at all periods of the treatment the thorough integration of these attitudes with existing dynamics is of paramount importance. Failing this the therapist runs the risk of falling back to the level of the primitive medicine man or the faith-healer and miracle-monger of our day. On the other hand there can be little doubt that persistent therapeutic failures sometimes seen in a highly trained analyst may be due to his inability to mobilize inner resources on the *psi* level: to integrate *psi* factors with clinical knowledge and acquired professional skills.

That the third period of treatment as it is envisaged here must make allowance for conflicts arising on the ego level goes without saying. Indeed, failing to pay due attention to intellectual, religious, and other ideological problems would leave the work of deep therapy incomplete. Paul Schilder[110a] has rightly pointed out that psychotherapy has to be as concerned with ideas, opinions, and ideologies as with other aspects of personality. He deplores the fact that psychoanalysis has "erected an artificial barrier between the so-called intellectual and the emotional sides of life." In this respect the Adlerian approach has provided a significant shift of emphasis from the original analytic position. The same tendency is reflected in the work of H. S. Sullivan,[125] Erich Fromm,[46] and in such neo-Adlerian departures from the Freudian school as that represented by Karen Horney[56] and her followers. It has specifically been emphasized by C. G. Jung.[65d]

All this shows once more that the part played by *psi* factors in the psychoanalytic situation cannot but be limited. It certainly must not detract from the importance of a primarily rational orientation of our approach to the patient. We must not forget that whatever be the potential telepathic effect of the analyst's unconscious therapeutic motivations they can only be brought to bear upon his patients on the basis of his full dynamic understanding of the existing clinical problem. Without such guidance he will grope in the dark like a surgeon who operates on his patient ignorant of the elementary facts of anatomy, relying only on the dim light of his intuition. Proper appreciation of *psi* undoubtedly serves as an important adjunct of psychoanalysis. However, such an advocate of the intuitive approach as Theodore Reik[101a] has rightly stated that "our unconscious feelers are there not to master a problem but to search for it." Our ultimate objective must be the integration of techniques congenial to the three principal aspects of the total personality conceived as part of a larger interpersonal "configuration."

* * *

How is a three-level approach along these lines likely to affect the practice of psychotherapy? What are the repercussions that can be expected in the immediate future? First and foremost, it is bound to modify the current "isolationist" or ivory-tower concept of the treatment situation itself. Our observations supplied ample evidence that the doctor-patient relationship can no longer be considered in terms of what John Rickman[105] described as a two-body problem. Even in the seclusion of the analyst's office the two are exposed to a ceaseless barrage of heteropsychic influences impinging upon them from their social environment and from the general cultural setting in which they are embedded. It is never the individual patient alone who lies on the therapist's couch. Invariably his friends and relations and a long line of ancestors are arraigned behind him and are involved in the treatment situation. Up to recently it has been common practice to pay attention to genealogical aspects—especially to hereditary traits that have been handed down to the patient from his forebears in the *perspective of time*. But we must realize that he may be equally affected by the interlacing patterns of illness and neurotic conflict that plague his next of kin, his friends and enemies *here* and *now*, in the *perspective of space*. Such examples of neurotic interaction as were discussed in Chapters XIV and XV have to be viewed against this broader background of multi-dimensional interpersonal relationships. They should go far to show that, as a matter of basic principle, mental or neurotic disorder is not confined to one isolated member of a family group. Like an ink-blot on blotting paper it tends to spread in all directions—in the perspective of both time and space. In the last analysis it is indicative of a disturbance in the interpersonal field at large and therefore calls for therapeutic action extending far beyond the confines of the individual or the family group. Paraphrasing a much-quoted saying of the inter-war period it could be stated: mental health, like peace, is indivisible—and so is war, neurosis, mental disorder, and human suffering in general.

For obvious reasons individual psychotherapy cannot be expected to do more than make a minimal dent in the fabric of society afflicted in such a way. But we have reason to believe that, however limited its immediate impact may be, it is apt to have far-reaching repercussions upon a wider circle of the patient's friends and relations and ultimately upon society at large. We must assume that the *psi* factor involved in the psychoanalytic situation operates in both directions. If doctor and patient are affected by their social environment, so is their social environment by whatever changes are effected in the treatment situation. The well-known example of a child's behaviour difficulties subsiding with improvement of his mother's condition is a case in point. A striking case of this type was described in Chapter XV. It stands for a great number of similar, though less striking, observations that occur in the practice of every experienced therapist.

It is interesting to note in this connection that H. S. Sullivan's[125] concept of mental illness as the result of disturbed interpersonal relationships is closely related to our thesis. So is the rationale of J. L. Moreno's[84a] sociometric approach. So, indeed, are all attempts at an organized attack on mental and neurotic disorder on the broader front of group therapy. All these recent developments reflect a new concept of the tasks of psychotherapy. They indicate that the therapist is no longer satisfied with confining his attention to the individual patient and his intrapsychic conflict. This is also one of the principal conclusions that have to be drawn from our approach. If the sick individual is but an integral part of a bigger bio-social configuration afflicted by disease psychotherapy must aim at changing the disturbed configuration as a whole. One could say: *It must aim at effecting the greatest degree of desirable change in the greatest number of people, conducive to the better functioning of society as a whole.*

Whether any one of the newly developed methods of group therapy, psychodrama, sociodrama, or what not, availing itself of the insight gained into *psi* factors, will bring us closer to this objective remains to be seen. Evidently there is no final solution to the problem and any sectarian approach can make but a small contribution towards it. But whatever the future holds in store it may be well to realize that in the last analysis success or failure of any method of psychotherapy does not solely depend on the scientific orientation and the professional skill of the individual therapist. It is equally dependent on the scope and power of the mandate society has given to him—and on the culturally determined limitations which are attached to his mandate. Both the individual and the group can only be reached by that kind of psychotherapy to which they are ready to submit. It cannot be brought to bear in an atmosphere of resistance nor even indifference. This is particularly true of an approach which presupposes the loosening of barriers separating the individual from *psi* aspects of his personality. Whether or not three-level therapy as conceived here will be permitted to have an impact, however feeble, upon our existing culture will ultimately be decided by the capacity of Western man to draw upon inner resources which for centuries past have been subject to repression, and to mobilize them in a determined effort at self-improvement.

BIBLIOGRAPHY

1. ABRAHAM, K.: A short study of the development of the libido viewed in the light of mental disorder. *Selected Papers*, New York, 1942.
2. ADLER, A.: *The Neurotic Constitution*, New York, 1917.
2a. *The Practice and Therapy of Individual Psychology*, Routledge & Kegan Paul, London, 1929.
3. ALEXANDER, F., and FRENCH, T. M.: *Studies in Psychosomatic Medicine*, Ronald Press, New York, 1948.
3a. *Psychosomatic Medicine*, Allen & Unwin, London, 1952.
4. ALLEE, W. C.: *Co-operation Among Animals*, Schuman, New York, 1951.
5. AMES, A.: quoted from: Ittleson and Kilpatrick in *Scientific American*, Aug. 1951.
6. AZAM, E.: *Hypnotism*, Paris, 1887.
7. BAIN: quoted from: Szondi: *Schicksalsanalyse*, Basle, 1948.
8. BENDER, H.: The case of Ilga K. Report of a phenomenon of unusual perception. *J. Parapsych.*, 2, 1938.
9. BENEDEK, T.: The psychosomatic implications of the primary unit: Mother-child. *Am. J. Orthopsychiat.*, 19, 1949.
10. BERGLER, E.: *Divorce Won't Help*, Harper Bros., New York, 1948.
11. BLEULER, E.: *Dementia Praecox or the Group of Schizophrenias*. Intern. Univ. Press, New York, and Allen & Unwin, London, 1950.
12. BOOTH, G.: Papers read to the Medical Section, Amer. Soc. Psych. Res., 1948–1951.
13. BRAMWELL, J. M.: *Hypnotism, Its History, Practice and Theory*, London, 1903.
14. BROAD, C. D.: The implications of psychical research, *J. Amer. Soc. Psych. Res.*, 41, 1947.
15. BRUGMANS, H. J. F. W.: *Une communication sur des expériences telepathic au laboratoire de psychologie à Groningen, etc.*, Premier Congr. Internat. des Res. Psychiques, 1922.
16. BUCK, A. E.: *Group Psychology and Therapy*. The Guild of Pastoral Psychology, Guild Lecture 56.
17. BURLINGHAM, D.: Child analysis and the mother, *Psychoan. Quart.*, 4, 1935.
18. CARINGTON, W.: *Telepathy, An Outline of its Facts, Theory and Implications*, Methuen & Co., London, 1947.

19. CARREL, A.: Physiological Time, *Science*, 74, 1931.
20. CHARI, C. T. K.: A note on precognition, *J. Amer. Soc. Psych. Res.*, 46, 1952.
21. CLEUGH, M. C.: *Time and its Importance in Modern Thought*, London, 1937.
22. COOPER, L. F., and ERICKSON, M. H.: Time distortion in hypnosis, *Bull. Georgetown Univ. Med. Cent.*, 1, 1948; ibid., 4, 1950.
23. COOLEY, C. H.: *Sociological Theory and Social Research*, New York, 1922.
24. COTTRELL, L. J., and DYMOND, R. F.: The empathic responses, a neglected field of research, *Psychiatry*, 12, 1949.
25. DARWIN, CH.: *The Origin of Species by Means of Natural Selection*, 1859.
26. DEUTSCH, H.: *The Psychology of Women*, Grune & Stratton, New York, 1944.
27. DEVEREUX, G.: Some criteria for the timing of confrontations and interpretations, *Int. J. Psychoan.*, 32, 1951.
28. DRAKE, R. M.: An unusual case of ESP, *J. Parapsych.*, 2, 1938.
29. DRIESCH, H.: *Science and Philosophy of the Organism*, London, 1908.
30. DUNBAR, F.: Effect of the mother's emotional attitude on the infant, *Psychosomatic Medicine*, 6, 1944.
31. DUNNE, J. W.: *An Experiment with Time*, Faber & Faber, London, 1927.
32. EHRENWALD, J.: *Telepathy and Medical Psychology*, Allen & Unwin, London, 1947; W. W. Norton, New York, 1948.
32*a*. Gibt es einen Zeitsinn? *Klin. Wschr.*, 10, 1931.
32*b*. Stoerung der Zeitauffassung der raumlichen und zeitlichen Orientierung des Zeichnens and des Rechnens bei einem Hirnverletzten, *Zschr. f. d. ges. Neur. u. Psych.*, 132, 1931.
32*c*. Hirnpathologische Bemerkungen zu einem Falle von "paranormalen" Erscheinungen bei einem Kinde (F. v. Neureiter), *Zschr. f. d. ges Neur. u. Psych.*, 157, 1937.
32*d*. Psychopathological aspects of telepathy, *Proc. Brit. Soc. Psych. Res.*, 1940.
32*e*. Quest for "psychics" and "psychical" phenomena in psychiatric studies of personality, *Psychiatr. Quart.*, 23, 1949.
32*f*. Telepathy in Dreams, *Brit. J. Med. Psychol.*, 20, 1944.
33. EISENBUD, J.: Telepathy and problems of psychoanalysis, *Psychoan. Quart.*, 15, 1946.
33*a*. Analysis of a presumptively telepathic dream, *Psychiat. Quart.*, 22, 1948.

33*b*. EISENBUD, J.: The dreams of two patients in analysis interpreted as a telepathic *rêve à deux*, *Psychoan. Quart.*, 16, 1947.

33*c*. Psychiatric contributions to parapsychology: a review, *J. Parapsych.*, 13, 1949.

33*d*. The use of the telepathy hypothesis in psychotherapy, in: *Specialized Techniques of Psychotherapy*, ed. Bychowski and Despert, Basic Books, New York, 1952.

33*e*. Papers read to the Medical Section of the Amer. Soc. Psych. Res., 1948–1950.

34. ELLIS, A.: Telepathy and psychoanalysis: a critique of recent "findings," *Psychiat. Quart.*, 21, 1947.

34*a*. Re-analysis of an alleged telepathic dream, *Psychiat. Quart.*, 23, 1949. (See also ibid.: replies by Eisenbud, Pederson-Krag, and Fodor.)

35. ERICKSON, M. H., and KUBIE, L. S.: The successful treatment of a case of acute hysterical depression, etc., *Psychiat. Quart.*, 10, 1941.

35*a*. The permanent relief of an obsessional phobia by means of communication with an unsuspected anal personality, *Psychoan. Quart.*, 8, 1939.

36. ESTABROOKS, G. H.: A contribution to experimental telepathy, *Boston Soc. Psych. Res. Bull.*, 5, 1927.

37. FENICHEL, O.: *The Psychoanalytic Theory of Neuroses*, W. W. Norton, New York, and Routledge & Kegan Paul, London, 1945.

38. FODOR, N.: Telepathy in analysis, *Psychiat. Quart.*, 21, 1947.

39. FOREL, A.: *Hypnotism or Suggestion and Psychotherapy*, New York, 1907.

40. FRANK, J.: Some aspects of lobotomy (prefrontal leukotomy) under psychoanalytic scrutiny. *Psychiatry*, 13, 1950.

41. FRANK, L. K., HUTCHINSON, G. E., LIVINGSTON, W. H., MCCULLOCH, W. S., and WIENER, N.: *Teleological Mechanisms*, Annals of the New York Academy of Sciences, 1948.

42. FRAZER, J. G.: *The Golden Bough*, Macmillan, London, 1890.

43. FRENCH, TH.: *The Integration of Behavior*, Univ. of Chicago Press, 1952.

44. FREUD, S.: *New Introductory Lectures on Psychoanalysis*, Hogarth Press, London, 1933.

44*a*. *The Interpretation of Dreams*, Allen & Unwin, London, 1925.

44*b*. *Psychopathology of Everyday Life*, Ernest Benn, London, 1924.

44*c*. FREUD, S.: Fragments of the analysis of a case of hysteria, *Coll. Papers*, Vienna, 1924.

44*d*. *The Ego and the Id*, Hogarth Press, London, 1923.

44*e*. *An Outline of Psychoanalysis*, Hogarth Press, London, and W. W. Norton, New York, 1949.

44*f*. *Totem and Taboo*, in Basic Writings of Sigmund Freud, Modern Library, New York, 1938, and Routledge & Kegan Paul, London.

44*g*. Mourning and melancholia, *Coll. Papers*, Vienna, 1924.

44*h*. *Three Contributions to the Theory of Sex*, New York and Washington, 1910, and Imago Publishing Co., London.

44*i*. Advice to the physician regarding psychoanalyic treatment, *Coll. Papers*, Vienna, 1925.

45. FRIES, J. F.: quoted from G. Murphy (86*b*).

46. FROMM, E.: *Escape from Freedom*, Rinehart, New York, 1947.

47. FROMM-REICHMAN, F.: Schizophrenia, in: *Specialized Techniques in Psychotherapy*, ed. Bychowski and Despert, Basic Books, 1952.

48. GELB, A., and GOLDSTEIN, K.: Psychologische Analysen hirnpathologischer Faelle, *Zschr. f. d. ges. Neur. u. Psych.*, 41, 1918.

49. GERSTMAN, J.: Fingeragnosie und isolierte Agraphie, *Zschr. f. d. ges. Neur. u. Psych.*, 108, 1927.

50. GLOVER, E.: *Freud or Jung*, Allen & Unwin, London, and W. W. Norton, New York, 1950.

51. GOLDSTEIN, K.: *The Organism*, American Book Co., New York, 1939.

52*a*. GILLESPIE, W. H.: Extrasensory elements in dream interpretation, in: *Psychoanalysis and the Occult*. Ed: G. Devereux, Intern. Univ. Press, New York, 1953.

52. GURNEY, E., MYERS, F. W. H., and PODMORE, F.: *Phantasms of the Living*, London, 1918.

53. HARTMAN, H., and KRIS, E.: Formation of psychic structure, in: *Psychoanalytic Study of the Child*, 2, New York, 1949.

54. HEAD, H.: *Aphasia and Kindred Disorders of Speech*, Macmillan, New York, and Cambridge University Press, London, 1926.

55. HOAGLAND, H.: The physiological control of judgements of duration; evidence for a chemical clock, *J. Gen. Psych.*, 9, 1933.

56. HORNEY, K.: *The Neurotic Personality of our Time*, W. W. Norton, New York, and Routledge & Kegan Paul, London, 1937.

57. HUBBARD, R. L.: *Dianetics*, Hermitage House, New York, 1950.

58. HUMPHREY, B.: Success in ESP related to form of response drawings: clairvoyance experiments, *J. Parapsych.*, 10, 1946.

59. ISENSCHMID, R.: Ueber die Wirkung der die Koerpertemperatur beeinflussenden Gifte auf Tiere ohne Waermeregulation, *Arch. f. Exp. Path.*, 75, 1913.

60. ITTLESON, W. H., and KILPATRICK, F. P.: *Scientific American*, Aug. 1951.

61. JAMES, W.: *The Principles of Psychology*, 1890.

62. JANET, P., and GILBERT: quoted from Eisenbud (33*c*).

63. JEPHSON, I.: Evidence for clairvoyance in card guessing, *Proc. Soc. Psych. Res.*, 38, 1928.

64. JOAD, C. E. M.: Book review in *New Statesman and Nation*, 23, 1948.

65. JUNG, C. G.: *Contributions to Analytical Psychology*, Harcourt, Brace & Co., New York, and Routledge & Kegan Paul, London, 1928.

65*a*. *The Integration of the Personality*, Farrar & Rinehart, New York, 1939, and Routledge & Kegan Paul, London, 1940.

65*b*. *The Psychology of Dementia Praecox*, Nerv. and Ment. Disorders Monograph Series, 1936.

65*c*. *Psychological Types*, etc., Harcourt, Brace & Co., New York, and Routledge & Kegan Paul, London, 1923.

65*d*. *Modern Man in Search of a Soul*, Routledge & Kegan Paul, London, 1944.

66. KAHN, D., and NEISSER, U. R.: (personal communication).

67. KANT, I.: *Traeume eines Geistersehers*, 1766.

68. KARDINER, A.: *The Psychological Frontiers of Society*, New York, 1945.

68*a*. Psychodynamics and the social sciences, in: *Culture and Personality*, Viking Fund, New York, 1949.

69. KLUCKHOHN, C., and MURRAY, H. A.: *Personality in Nature, Society and Culture*, Knopf & Co., New York, 1949.

70. KOEHLER, W.: *Gestalt Psychology*, Liveright, New York, 1947.

71. KRETSCHMER, E.: *Physique and Character*, Routledge and Kegan Paul, London, 1925.

72. KROPOTKIN, P.: *Mutual Aid, a Factor in Evolution*, Knopf & Co., New York, 1914.

73. LEVINE, M.: Principles of psychiatric treatment, in: *Dynamic Psychiatry*, ed. Alexander and Ross, 1952.

74. LIPPS, TH.: *Raumaesthetik und geometrisch optische Taeuschungen*, 1897.

75. LITTLE, M.: Counter-transference and the patient's response to it, *Int. J. Psychoan.*, 32, 1951.
76. LOEWENSTEIN, R.: The problem of interpretation, *Psychoan. Quart.*, 20, 1951.
77. MACH, E.: *Analyse der Empfindungen*, Jena, 1906.
78. MASSERMAN, I.: *Principles of Dynamic Psychiatry*, Saunders, New York, 1946.
79. MCCLEARY, R., and LAZARUS, R. S.: Autonomic discrimination without awareness: an interim report, *J. Personality*, 18, 1949.
80. MEAD, G. H.: *Mind, Self and Society*, Univ. of Chicago Press, 1934.
81. MEERLOO, J.: Telepathy as a form of archaic communication *Psychiat. Quart.*, 23, 1949.
81*a*. *Patterns of Panic*, Internat. Univ. Press, New York, 1950.
81*b*. *Conversation and Communication*, Internat. Univ. Press, 1953.
81*c*. Papers read to the Medical Section, Amer. Soc. Psych. Res., 1948–1951.
82. MITCHELL, T. W.: *Medical Psychology and Psychical Research*, London, 1922.
83. MITTELMANN, B.: Marital problems, in: *Specialized Techniques in Psychotherapy*, ed. Bychowski & Despert, Basic Books, 1952.
84. MORENO, J. L.: *Who Shall Survive?* New York, 1934.
84*a*. *Group-Psychotherapy*, New York, 1945.
85. MULLAHY, P.: *Oedipus, Myth and Complex*, Hermitage Press, New York, and Allen & Unwin, London, 1948.
86. MURPHY, G., ROSS, O. A., and SCHMEIDLER, G. R.: The spontaneity factor in extrasensory perception, *J. Am. Soc. Psych. Res.*, 46, 1952.
86*a*. MURPHY, G.: Psychical phenomena and human needs, *J. Amer. Soc. Psych. Res.*, 37, 1943.
86*b*. *Historical Introduction to Modern Psychology*, Harcourt, Brace & Co., New York, 1949, and Routledge & Kegan Paul, London.
86*c*. MURPHY, G., and NEWCOMB, T. M.: *Experimental Social Psychology, An Interpretation of Research upon the Socialization of the Individual*, New York, 1937.
87. MYERS, F. W. H.: *Human Personality and its Survival of Bodily Death*, London, 1903.
88. NEUREITER, F. V.: *Wissen um fremdes Wissen, auf unbekanntem Wege erworben*, Gotha, 1935.
89. NÖUY, LECOMTE DE: *Human Destiny*, New York, 1947.

90. OBERNDORF, C. P.: Psychoanalysis of married couples, *Psychoan. Review*, 25, 1938.

91. OVERSTREET, H. A.: *The Mature Mind*, W. W. Norton, New York, 1949, and Gollancz, London, 1950.

92. PEARSON, K.: quoted from: Szondi: *Schicksalsanalyse*, Basle, 1948.

93. PEDERSON-KRAG, G.: Telepathy and repression, *Psychoan. Quart.*, 6, 1947.

93*a*. Papers read to the Medical Section, Amer. Soc. Psych. Res., 1948–1951.

94. PLATO: *Symposion.*

95. POETZL, O., and HOFF, H.: *Zschr. f. d. ges. Neur. u. Psych.*, 151, 1934.

96. PRATT, J. G., and WOODRUFF, I. L.: Size of stimulus symbols in extrasensory perception, *J. Parapsychol.*, 3, 1939.

97. RANK, O.: *Will Therapy, Truth and Reality*, Knopf & Co., New York, 1947.

97*a*. *The Trauma of Birth*, Harcourt, Brace & Co., New York, 1929.

98. REGARDIE, F. J.: Analysis of a homosexual, *Psychiat. Quart.*, 23, 1949.

99. REICH, A.: On counter-transference, *Int. J. Psychoan.*, 32, 1951.

100. REICH, W.: *Character Analysis*, Orgone Institute Press, New York, 1949.

101. REIK, TH.: *A Psychologist Looks at Love*, Rinehart & Co., New York, 1944.

101*a*. *Listening with the Third Ear*, Farrar Strauss, New York, 1948, and Allen & Unwin, London, 1950 (as *Inner Experiences of a Psychoanalyst*).

102. RENOLDS, A. E., *et al.*: Reactions of the adrenal gland to physical and emotional stress in college oarsmen, *New England J. Med.*, 244, 1951.

103. RHINE, J. B.: *The Reach of the Mind*, W. Sloane, New York, 1947, and Faber & Faber, London, 1948.

103*a*. RHINE, J. B., PRATT, J. G., SMITH, B. H., STUART, C. E., and GREENWOOD, J. A.: *Extrasensory Perception after Sixty Years*, New York, 1940.

103*b*. RHINE, J. B.: Telepathy and clairvoyance reconsidered with comment by W. Carington, I. Hettinger, R. H. Thouless, G. N. M. Tyrell, C. D. Broad, and Denys Parsons, *Proc. Soc. Psych. Res.*, 48, 1946.

103c. RHINE, J. B., and HUMPHREY, B. M.: The PK effect: special evidence from hit patterns, first quarter distribution of the page, *J. Parapsych.*, 8, 1944.

104. RICHET, CH.: *Proc. Soc. Psych. Res.*, 6, 1889.

105. RICKMAN, J.: The factor of numbers in individual and group dynamics, *J. Ment. Science*, 96, 1950.

106. RÓHEIM, G.: Psychoanalysis and anthropology, in: *Psychoanalysis Today*, ed. S. Lorand, New York, 1933, and Allen & Unwin, London, 1949.

106a. *Animism, Magic and the Divine King*, New York, 1930.

107. RUESCH, J., and BATESON, G.: *Communication*, W. W. Norton, New York, 1951.

108. RUSSELL, B.: *Human Knowledge, Its Scope and Limits*, Allen & Unwin, London, and Simon & Schuster, New York, 1948.

109. SALTMARSH, H. F.: Report on cases of apparent precognition, *Proc. Soc. Psych. Res.*, 42, 1934.

110. SCHILDER, P.: *Imago*, 20, 1934.

110a. *Psychotherapy*, W. W. Norton, New York, 1938.

110b. *Psychoanalysis, Man and Society*, W. W. Norton, New York, 1951.

111. SCHMEIDLER, G. R.: Predicting good and bad scores in a clairvoyance experiment: a final report, *J. Am. Soc. Psych. Res.*, 37, 1943.

112. SERVADIO, E.: Psychoanalysis and Telepathy, *Imago*, 21, 1935.

113. SCHROEDINGER, E.: *What is Life?* Cambridge University Press, London, 1944, and Macmillan, New York, 1946.

114. SHERIF, M.: quoted from: Murphy (86*b*).

115. SIMMEL, E.: The "Doctor Game," illness and the profession of medicine, in: *The Psychoanalytic Reader*, ed. R. Fliess, Internat. Univ. Press, New York, 1948.

116. SINCLAIR, U.: *Mental Radio*, New York, 1930.

117. SKINNER, B. F.: *Science and Human Behavior*, Macmillan, New York, 1953.

118. SOAL, S. G., and GOLDNEY, K. M.: Experiments in precognitive telepathy, *Proc. Soc. Psych. Res.*, 47, 1943.

118a. SOAL, S. G.: *The Experimental Situation in Psychical Research.* 9th Myers Memorial Lecture, London, 1947.

119. SPENCER, H.: *Principles of Psychology*, 1853.

120. SPERLING, M.: Analysis of a case of recurrent ulcer of the leg, in: *Psychoanalytic Study of the Child*, 3, New York, 1949.

120a. Children's interpretation and reaction to the unconscious of their mothers, *Internat. J. Psychoan.*, 31, 1950.

121. SPITZ, R., and WOLF, K. M.: Autoerotism, some empirical findings and hypotheses on three of its manifestations in the first year of life, in: *Psychoanalytic Study of the Child*, 3, New York, 1949.

122. ST. FRANCIS OF SALE: quoted from *Year of Grace*, Gollancz, London, 1950, and Houghton Mifflin, Boston, 1951 (under title *Man and God*).

123. STORCH, A.: *The Primitive Archaic Forms of Inner Experience and Thought in Schizophrenics*, Nerv. and Mental Disorders Monograph Series, 1924.

124. STRAUSS, B. V.: The role of the physician's personality in medical practice. (Psychotherapeutic Medicine), *New York State J. Med.*, 51, 1951.

125. SULLIVAN, H. S.: *Conceptions of Modern Psychiatry*, Washington, D.C., 1947.

126. SZONDI, L.: *Schicksalsanalyse*, Basle, 1948.

127. SZUREK, S. A., and JOHNSON, A. M.: The genesis of antisocial acting out in children and adults, *Psychoan. Quart.*, 21, 1952.

128. TILLICH, P.: *The Protestant Era*, Univ. of Chicago Press, 1948.

129. THOULESS, R. H.: Thought transference and related phenomena, *Proc. Royal Instit. Great Britain*, 34, 1951.

129*a*. THOULESS, R. H., and WIESNER, B. P.: The *psi* processes in normal and "paranormal" psychology, *J. Parapsych.*, 12, 1948.

130. TOYNBEE, A.: *A Study of History*, Oxford Univ. Press, London and New York, 1946.

131. TYRELL, G. N. M.: *Science and Psychical Phenomena*, New York, 1939.

132. UEXKUELL, J. V.: *Umwelt und Innenwelt der Tiere*, Berlin, 1921.

133. ULLMAN, M.: Communication, *J. Am. Soc. Psych. Res.*, 42, 1948.

133*a*. On the nature of resistance to *psi* experiences, *J. Am. Soc. Psych. Res.*, 46, 1952.

133*b*. Papers read to the Medical Section, Amer. Soc. Psych. Res., New York, 1948–1951.

134. USHER, F. L., and BURT, F. P.: Thought transference, *Annals of Psychic Science*, 8, 1909.

134*a*. URBAN, H. J.: Parapsychologie und Psychiatrie, *Poetzl Festschrift*, Wagner, Innsbruck, 1946.

134*b*. *Psi* in Psychiatrie, *Deutsche Med. Rundschau*, 3, 1949.

135. WARCOLLIER, R.: *Mind to Mind*, Creative Age Press, New York, 1948.

135*a*. *Experimental Telepathy*, Boston, 1938.

136. WHEELER, W. M.: *Social Life Among Insects*, Harcourt Brace & Co., New York, 1923, and Routledge & Kegan Paul, London, 1928.
137. WOLBERG, R. L.: *Hypnoanalysis*, Grune & Stratton, New York, 1945.
138. ZULLIGER, H.: Prophetic Dreams, *Internat. Zschr. f. Psychoan*, 18, 1932.

GLOSSARY

of unusual and equivocal terms

AGENT: In tests for telepathy, the person whose mental states are to be apprehended by the percipient.

ANAPSYCHIC: Pertaining to the building-up phase of mental metabolism, comparable to the anabolic or building-up phase of chemical metabolism.

A-PATHIC: Lacking of empathy.

AUTOPSYCHE: The mind of oneself.

CATAPSYCHIC: Pertaining to the phase of disorganization or breakdown in mental metabolism, comparable to the catabolic phase of chemical metabolism.

CLAIRVOYANCE: Extrasensory perception of objective events as distinguished from telepathic perception of the mental or subjective events of another person.

EMPATHY: The imaginative projection of one person into another person's consciousness.

EMPATHIC AGNOSIA: Lack of empathic responsiveness, comparable to sensory aphasia.

ENKINESIS: The motor counterpart of empathy; the imaginative projection of one person into another person's motor, psychomotor or glandular behaviour.

ESP (Extrasensory Perception): Response to an external event not presented to any known sense.

HETEROPSYCHE: Another person's mind.

LOCALIZATION, PLURI-CEREBRAL: The theory which assumes that potentially a person's mental processes may be "localized" in more than one person's central nervous system or in "brain regions" scattered in space.

LOCALIZATION, UNI-CEREBRAL: The theory which assumes that a person's mental functions are exclusively "localized" in his central nervous system, particularly in his brain.

MEDIUM: A person subject to mental dissociation amounting to trance states which are claimed to favour the origin of psychic phenomena.

METALOGICAL: A conceptual scheme disregarding the familiar categories or modes of thinking in terms of time, space, and causality. *Psi* phenomena are part of a metalogical series, by contrast to mechanistic and teleological series studied by the physicist or the introspectionist psychologist respectively. Metalogical series are not illogical nor irrational but have a logic of their own and are subject to the laws of psychodynamics.

PARAPSYCHOLOGY: A division of psychology dealing with those psychical effects which appear not to fall within the scope of what is at present recognized law.

PERCIPIENT: The person who makes the call in ESP tests or who apprehends the mental states of one agent under spontaneous conditions.

PRECOGNITION: Cognition of a future event which could not be known through rational inference.

PSI: A general term to identify personal factors or processes in nature which transcend accepted laws but are subject to familiar psychodynamic principles. It is close to the popular use of the word "psychic" and the technical one "parapsychical."

PSI LEVEL OF FUNCTIONING: That level or area of the psychic apparatus which is primarily concerned with *psi* functions, by contrast to the ego and id levels. There is, however, a considerable area of overlapping of *psi* and id levels.

PSI PHENOMENA: Occurrences which result from the operation of *psi*. They include the phenomena of both ESP (including precognition) and PK.

PSYCHO-KINETIC EFFECT (PK): The direct influence exerted on a physical system by a subject without any known intermediate energy or instrumentation.

PSYCHO-MITOSIS: The conflict involving the psychological separation of parent and child, comparable to cell division or mitosis in the life cycle of a cell. The conflict of psycho-mitosis precedes the Oedipal conflict.

SIGNIFICANCE, PSYCHOLOGICAL: The meaningful nature of a suggested interpretation, helping to fill a gap in the dynamic understanding of a given psychological situation failing which the situation would remain unintelligible.

SIGNIFICANCE, STATISTICAL: A numerical result is significant if it equals or surpasses some criterion of degree of chance improbability. Common criteria are: a probability value of 0·01 or less, or a deviation in the expected direction such that the critical ratio is 2·33 or greater.

TELEPATHY: Extrasensory perception of the mental activities of another person. It does not include the clairvoyant perception of objective events.

TRACER EFFECT: The appearance of well-defined identifying data or of a multiplicity of distinctive features in mental content presumed to be telepathic.

TRACER ELEMENTS: Cognitive or ideational elements permitting such identification, e.g. in the manifest content of a dream.

Definitions of technical terms used in the literature of psychical research are quoted from a Glossary appended to numbers of the *Journal of Parapsychology*, Duke University Press, Durham, N. C., edited by J. B. Rhine and Associates. The responsibility for other definitions used is largely my own.

Index